Chiropractic:
The Miracle Within

In memory of Dr. Sid Williams,

Founder of Life Chiropractic College
and Life University

by Fran Addeo, D.C.

Frantastic Books are available through Ingram Press,
and available for order through Ingram Press Catalogues

A Frantastic Books LLC book Published by Create Space,
a division of Amazon

Disclaimer

The information contained in this book should not be used
to self-diagnose or treat any condition and is no substitute for
professional healthcare.
The author does not accept responsibility for any adverse effects
resulting from the use of any idea, suggestion, or information
contained in this book. Always consult with your medical doctor or
chiropractor before stopping, starting, or changing your healthcare
program.

Visit my website DrFranAddeo.com

Printed in the United States of America

First Printing, January 2014

Frantastic Books, LLC

Paperback ISBN 978-1-62747-047-6

Ebook ISBN 978-1-62747-048-3

Special Thanks

Dr. Phil VanAllsburg
for your help in creating the concept for this book

Sue Tompkins and Lisa Addeo Colen
for your editing suggestions

Table of Contents

Preface
Definition of a Miracle   xi
The Philosophy of Chiropractic   xi
Universal Intelligence   xii
Innate Intelligence   xii

Chapter 1
My Story
Why I Became a Chiropractor   1
Subluxations   3
A Piece of the Health-Care Puzzle   5

Chapter 2
Various Chiropractic Techniques
Manual Manipulation   7
The Activator Method   8

Chapter 3
ADIO
Requirements for Chiropractic College   14
Above, Down, Inside, Out   16
New Humans   17
Interference to Innate   20

Chapter 4
Subluxations—the Silent Killer
Subluxation Defined 21
Bone Component 22
Nerve Component 22
Muscular Component 23
The Soft Tissue Component 23
Chemical Component 23

Chapter 5
Believe It or Not
"I'll Give You One Shot" 27
Alyson's Miracle 28

Chapter 6
Preventing Arthritis
Arthritis Defined 30
*Rick's Neck – X-rays before and after
adjustments 31*
The Limitation of Matter 36
It's My Sacroiliac – Stress on the Hip Joint 37

Chapter 7
Chiropractic for Children
Birth – The First Subluxation 39
Adjusting Babies 40
Scoliosis and the Little Cowgirl 42
A Shortage of Chiropractors? 45

Chapter 8
X-rays
History of X-rays   48
Some Chiropractic Techniques Require X-rays   51
The C1 Adjustment   54

Chapter 9
Cervical Spine (the Neck)
Atlas   56
Christopher Reeves   57
Bell's Palsy   59
Dizziness   60
Headaches   63
The "Stress Vertebra"   63
Nerve Supply to Thyroid Gland   64
Draining Waste from the Brain   65
Antioxidants   65
Head and Neck Exercises   66

Chapter 10
Thoracic Spine T1 – T12 (the Mid Back)
Nerve Supply to Lower Arms and Hands   69
Nerve Supply to Heart and Lungs   70
Nerve Supply to Gallbladder   72
Nerve Supply to Stomach and Liver   75
Diabetes and the Pancreas   75
The Immune System   78
Nerve Supply to Adrenal Glands   79
Nerve Supply to Kidneys   80
Nerve Supply to Fallopian Tubes   83

Infertility   83
The Golfer Guy   84

Chapter 11
Lumbar Spine (the Low Back)
Nerve Supply to Large Intestine   87
The Garden Hose Analogy   88
Nerve Supply to Knee   92
Pending Joint Replacements   93
Sciatica   95
The Prostate Gland   96
Articular Fixations – The "Miracle Cure"   97
Pain Is an Emotion   102

Chapter 12
The Pelvis and Sacrum
Robert the Architect   104
The Body Adapts to Subluxations   105
Lori's Lateral Sacrum   106

Chapter 13
The Extremities
TMJ – Jaw Pain   109
The Carpal Tunnel   110
Ted the Tennis Player   111
The Body Needs Time to Heal   112
Maintaining Mike's Machine   114
Childbirth and the Tailbone   114
Lower Legs and Feet   115

Plantar Fasciitis – Subluxation
of the Heel Bone   117

Chapter 14
Posture
Perfect Alignment   119
Ergonomics   120
Sitting Is the New Smoking   121
Forward Head Posture   122
Hold in Your Tummy   124
Watch Your Neck   125

Chapter 15
Stress Management
Nervous Tension   127
Grumpy Patients   130
Learning to Relax   130
Breathing and Stretching   132

Chapter 16
Food for Thought
The (SAD) Standard American Diet   134
Got Meat?   135
Meatless Mondays   137
Lab-Produced Meat   137
Food Choices   138
The Shellfish Story   139
GMOs   140

Chapter 17
Think for Yourself
*"Whatever You Do, Don't Go to a
Chiropractor!"   142*
"You Have to Keep Going Back"   144
*Stages of Care- Relief, Corrective and
Maintenance Care   145*
The Chiropractic Lifestyle   146

Chapter 18
Spinal Hygiene
Take Care of Your Spine   148
Ligaments, Muscles, and Tendons   149
Sprains and Strains   149
Tendonitis   150
Whatever You Do, No Heat!   150
Taking Care of the Adjustment   152
Laughter   155

Appendix
Chart of the Nervous System   157
Recommended Reading   158
Contact the Author   159

Preface

A miracle is defined as a surprising event that cannot be explained in normal or scientific terms, and is thought to be divine in nature.

As spiritual beings having a physical experience, humans try to explain and understand everything about the physical world in scientific terms. But some things, such as the miracle of life itself, cannot be explained. For instance, even though scientists have put a man on the moon, they cannot figure out how to create a living cell from the simple elements found in living tissue.

The human body has an amazing miracle within – a vital force that creates life and maintains health. From the moment a sperm and egg unite until the moment you take your last breath, this vital force is the miracle within you, controlling the beating of your heart and digesting the food you eat.

The Philosophy of Chiropractic

The philosophy of chiropractic is based on the idea that a Universal Intelligence is creating and guiding the physical world. The human body has an innate intelligence which allows our body to function, adapt, and heal.

Universal Intelligence

Universal Intelligence is a concept that is known by many different names. Many people call it God. Some call it source energy. Others feel more comfortable calling it infinite potential, the chi, the light, a higher power, love, or quantum field potential. Whatever word or term humans use to describe it, this Universal Intelligence, which is the backdrop to life on Earth, is a powerful force.

B.J. Palmer called this Universal Intelligence a cosmic power, a "mysterious something" that is behind all creation. He also referred to the Universal Intelligence as a "magic power" that transforms the food we eat into living, physical bodies and provides us with beautiful sunsets and flowers.

Innate Intelligence

The innate intelligence of the body maintains health by regulating temperature, blood pressure, respiratory rate, blood sugar level, and other functions of the body. The innate intelligence of the body is a vital force that can heal the body, as demonstrated by the mending of a broken bone or the healing of a cut on the skin.

The vital force of the body flows through the nervous system - from the brain, down the spinal cord, and out to every cell and organ of the body. This vital force allows the body to adapt, heal, and function from the moment of conception to the moment of death.

Chiropractors find and correct subtle misalignments of the bones, which are interfering with the flow of the vital force through the nerves of the body. A chiropractic adjustment removes the interference to this vital force and allows the miracle within to be experienced as healing and an improved sense of well-being.

Most people associate chiropractors with neck pain or back pain. However, chiropractic care ensures that the signals from the brain flow freely through the nervous system to maintain the health of the entire body.

Chapter One
My Story

The year was 1977. It was a rainy afternoon in Fort Lauderdale and I was driving home from work in rush-hour traffic. The cars ahead of me were stopping rather quickly, so I hit the brakes, and the next thing I knew, KABOOM! My car was hit from behind and forced into the car ahead of me. I suffered a whiplash injury and felt a little lightheaded, but I didn't want to go to the hospital. I wanted to go home and put a heating pad on my neck because I was already beginning to feel stiff and sore.

Years later, I learned that a heating pad was the worst thing I could have done. I didn't know that using ice for short periods of time was the best thing to do for injuries. I was young and unaware of many things, including chiropractic.

Like many people, I had no idea what chiropractors do, and I suffered needlessly for two years. My neck and upper back were stiff and sore, and the pain in my low back was shooting down my leg, making it impossible for me to enjoy doing the things I wanted to do, such as taking walks on the beach and going to the gym. So when all else failed, I took the advice of a friend and decided that it was time to try chiropractic.

At the time, I was working as a feature writer for the Fort Lauderdale News. For two years, from the time of my accident to my first visit to a chiropractor, I tried many different things in my quest for healing, and wrote newspaper stories about some of them. Different things work for different people, but nothing was working for me until I tried chiropractic.

Healing techniques, such as medications, physical therapy, acupuncture, massage, therapeutic exercises, ultrasound, electric stimulation of muscles, heat packs, ice packs, roller tables, vibrations stations, nutrition counseling, emotional release techniques, and injection of homeopathic and other pain-relieving substances, all have value for some people. But what I needed for my healing was a chiropractic adjustment.

As a chiropractor who has adjusted thousands of patients and seen thousands of miracles, both large and small, my goal in writing this book is to share what I know to be true. Chiropractic is a unique and powerful source of natural healing. Yet many people don't understand or know what it is that chiropractors do.

Some chiropractors offer many different treatments besides the chiropractic adjustment in their offices. Some offer massage, physical therapy treatments, nutrition counseling, and acupuncture. All of these are good and can help release the healing miracle within their patients.

However, the chiropractic adjustment should not be confused with other things that chiropractors do. What sets the chiropractic adjustment apart is that chiropractors are trained to find and correct subluxations.

Subluxations

A subluxation is a subtle misalignment of a bone in the skeletal system that causes interference to the flow of mental impulses that travel from the brain to every cell and organ of the body.

When a friend suggested I go see their chiropractor, I had no idea what to expect. During my first chiropractic visit, the chiropractor found that I had several subluxations. He explained to me how these bones had been jarred out of their proper position during the car crash and were causing interference to the nervous system. I learned that my subluxations were the cause of my pain and suffering.

Looking at the chart of the spinal column, I saw how the nerves come out from between the bones of the spinal column and travel to all the muscles and organs of the body. I understood how a minor misalignment of the bone would cause nerve interference and pain. It made perfect sense to me. Pinched nerves in my back and neck were the cause of my problems.

There was nothing unpleasant or uncomfortable about the adjustment, only relief from my pain and suffering.

"It's like getting your car aligned," he said, smiling. "Your vehicle will run much better now."

After my first adjustment, I couldn't believe how much better I felt. It was a miracle.

Looking back, I see that my car accident was a blessing in disguise. It changed the course of my life and led to me becoming a chiropractor myself.

I have been a chiropractor for more than twenty years, and like many chiropractors, after years of adjusting thousands of patients, I sometimes take miracles for granted. As one of my colleagues said, the miracles that chiropractors see every day are "miracles in the line of duty."

Chiropractic care is a mystery to many, even to patients who enjoy the benefit of chiropractic care.

"It's a miracle!" they say, getting off the adjusting table and realizing their headache is gone or their low back feels better even before leaving my office.

Whether it's on a "I'll call you when I need you" basis or "sign me up for a once a month checkup," chiropractic patients like getting their adjustments.

As a chiropractor, I believe there are miracles within us all, waiting to be expressed as improved health and sense of well-being. Chiropractic adjustments release the miracle within.

While working as a feature writer, I was required to present five story ideas to my editor every Monday morning. After a few years, it was challenging to come up with new ideas for stories. As a chiropractor, I never run out of good stories. Every new patient is another story that demonstrates the miracle within, and

I will be sharing many of these success stories with you in my book.

A Piece of the Health-Care Puzzle

There are many different healing techniques and different things work for different people. Sometimes, more than one thing is needed to release the miracle within. Many patients who make their way to chiropractic offices decide to try chiropractic as a last resort. Many times, chiropractic care is the answer to releasing the miracle within, even when all else has failed.

When these patients make their way to my office, I share my story with them, telling them how nothing worked for me until I gave chiropractic a try. I tell them that I was once in their shoes, without hope of ever regaining my health, and how I was so amazed at how much chiropractic helped me that I became a chiropractor myself. Then I find and correct the subluxations causing the interference so they can experience the miracle within.

As I will explain in this book, what chiropractors do is unique. No other health-care professional is trained to do what chiropractors do. I'm not saying that other health-care providers cannot release the miracles within their patients, because they can and they do. But different people respond differently to different healing techniques. When one thing doesn't bring forth the healing miracle within, another avenue should be considered.

In my practice, I refer my patients to other health professionals if I believe it will be beneficial. These include medical doctors, physical therapists, acupuncturists, and massage therapists.

Chiropractic care is an important piece of the health-care puzzle, and as I have seen in my practice, chiropractic adjustments can make the other healing techniques, including medication, more effective.

Chapter Two
Various Chiropractic Techniques

There are many different chiropractic techniques taught at chiropractic colleges. It is the personal choice of the chiropractic students to decide which technique or techniques they will use to adjust their patients.

Some techniques involve manual manipulation of the joints. These manual adjustments involve turning and twisting the joints of the spinal column. This type of adjustment gives an audible "popping" sound. The sound that is made during a chiropractic adjustment is the sound of synovial gas being released from the joint. It can be compared to the sound that is made when a bottle of champagne is opened.

There are other chiropractic techniques that involve applying a barely perceivable pressure. The technique that is used depends upon the individual chiropractor and the patient's preference. Some chiropractic patients prefer manual adjustments and others choose to go to chiropractors who use one of the many "light force" techniques that work just as well. I like to say "it's not the technique, it's the technician." It's simply a matter of personal preference.

As for me, I haven't twisted or popped or cracked or manipulated a joint since I was a student at Life Chiropractic College a quarter century ago. Even though I was taught how to do that, I never felt comfortable doing the manipulation style adjustment on others. It's not the way I like to get adjusted, so I was happy to learn, and happy to use, the Activator Method in my practices. It's easy on my patients and easy on me, and, like all chiropractic techniques, it can release the miracles within.

The Activator Method

The Activator Method is a very gentle, specific, light force chiropractic technique that involves no "popping" or "twisting" of the joints. The Activator adjustment is made with a handheld, spring-loaded mechanical instrument that delivers a high-speed, low-force tap through a rubber tip. The Activator Method uses a system of analysis involving leg length checks to determine the precise location where the adjustment is needed. The Activator adjusting instrument is then used to deliver a metered light force adjustment.

Dr. Arlan Fuhr, a leader of the chiropractic profession and cofounder of Activator Methods International, travels the world, teaching chiropractors how to use the Activator Method. Advanced proficiency rated Activator doctors, such as myself, are highly trained to use the Activator Method system of analysis to find and correct subluxations or minor misalignments that interfere with the flow of your vital life force.

While the thousands of patients I have adjusted using the Activator adjusting instrument have loved it and referred their friends and families to me, some people like the manual manipulation style of chiropractic adjustments. Some patients visit my office saying they need "a good crack" because their back or neck is stiff and sore. When I tell them that I don't do manual manipulation, they look at me questioningly. Then I show them my Activator adjusting instrument and explain to them that I can give a very good adjustment without popping or twisting. I tell them that research projects and clinical trials have shown that the Activator Method is just as effective as manual adjustments for correcting subluxations. Sometimes, they will give it a try, and other times, they won't.

"That won't work for me," they say, turning away. I refer these patients to a chiropractor who does manual adjustments. I think some people like to hear the popping sound and the feeling of getting the joints manually manipulated, but that is not the technique I prefer to use.

I also have chiropractors who refer patients to me who do not want the manual style of adjusting. These patients would not consider any chiropractic technique except for the Activator Method. Many patients tell me how skeptical they were that such a low-force, gentle adjustment could be so beneficial, and how pleasantly surprised they were that it worked so well for releasing the miracle within them.

It's good for you to know that there are many different types of chiropractic techniques out there. It's just a matter of finding a technique that appeals to you.

Chiropractors are known for helping patients with neck pain and back pain, but chiropractic adjustments do a lot more than just fix the pain in your neck and back. I will be sharing many success stories about the miracles released from within that helped all sorts of health problems, beginning with this story about one of my very first patients.

A woman came to see me complaining of a stiff neck. While talking with her and taking her case history, she told me that she had not been able to taste or smell for years.

"I won't let my husband take me out for dinner, even on our anniversary, because I can't smell or taste the food. To me, going out to dinner is just a waste of money," she said, somewhat sadly.

I made note of this in her file and proceeded to do my exam. I asked her to turn her head to the left and right. She could barely turn her head to the left or the right, and she said it hurt when she tried. She reported no recent trauma, but said she was sick and tired of the pain. After being urged to do so by a neighbor, she decided it was time to try a chiropractor.

Using the method of analysis in the Activator technique that I have been trained to use, I found that she had subluxations of C1 and C2, the two top bones in her neck. Interestingly, fifty percent of the rotation of the neck occurs at C1 and C2.

Her subluxation was preventing the normal rotation of her neck and exerting pressure on the nerves exiting between them. This was causing the pain and tenderness in the surrounding muscles.

The nervous system begins with the brain. The spinal cord is an extension of the brain. Every nerve in the body can be traced back to the base of the skull, where the spinal cord begins. Even the nerves in the knee, if traced back up through the nervous system, begin in the upper cervical spine. Because every nerve in the body starts at the base of the skull, where the brain becomes the spinal cord, some chiropractors believe that C1 and C2 are the most important subluxations that need to be corrected. (One of my professors at Life Chiropractic College told me that he knows his C1 is out of alignment when his right knee hurts!)

After telling my patient that I thought her neck pain was most likely a chiropractic problem that I could correct, and after explaining to her what I was going to do, with her permission, I used the Activator Method protocol of analysis to find the correct line of correction. Using the Activator adjusting instrument, I made the adjustment, which, to the patient, seemed like a little tap on C1 and a little tap on C2. A few other adjustments and her first adjustment was complete.

As I tell all of my patients, everyone is different and the number of adjustments needed to reach maximum improvement can vary from person to person. I suggest two or three visits before deciding if this is working. I told her that some people feel almost all better after one, two, or three visits, and others may need more.

If a patient does not respond to my care within a few visits, I refer them out for X-rays, making sure that they don't have a condition that requires immediate medical attention. Rarely the cause of the pain could be a tumor or infection or other underlying disease process. These problems are beyond the scope of chiropractic, and require evaluation and treatment by a medical doctor. Also, if I determine during my examination that theirs is not a chiropractic problem, I immediately refer them to a medical doctor, or even to the emergency room, if that is what I think they need.

My patient agreed with my recommended care plan and scheduled another appointment later that week. She came in smiling, saying that she was definitely feeling better, and we both could see that she could turn her head to the left and right much more easily. I adjusted her again and could tell that she wasn't out of alignment nearly as much, and this was good. We scheduled her third appointment for the following week.

When she showed up for her third appointment, I was a little concerned. She wasn't smiling. In fact, she had tears in her eyes.

"What is it?" I asked.

She could barely keep from crying. "I can smell. And I can taste," she said, wiping the tears from her eyes. "I was in the car with my husband and I could smell gasoline. When I told him that I could smell gas, he told me that he put the gas can for the lawnmower in the back of the vehicle because he needed to stop at the gas station and fill it. And then we were eating dinner, and I could taste the onions. It's a miracle!"

It was October and the holidays were just around the corner, and she had just one concern.

"I'm afraid that I am going to eat too much during the holidays and gain weight!"

Of course, she was joking and we laughed about what a lovely problem that was going to be.

Chapter Three
ADIO

When I decided to become a chiropractor, I felt that it was a "calling." It was something I just had to do. To this day, I feel I am on a mission to help others, as I was helped. I wanted to help people heal naturally, without drugs or surgery. Sharing chiropractic with as many people as I could would become the purpose of my life.

I had no idea what I was getting myself into when I took the first steps to entering Life Chiropractic College. Looking back, that was probably a good thing. Soon after making the decision to go back to school to become a chiropractor, I found out I would have to go back to college for two years to get the classes that were required for admission to chiropractic college. I majored in journalism and did not have any of the sciences that were required or the math that was needed to go along with them. Those classes included college-level anatomy, microbiology, chemistry, physics, algebra, and geometry.

Getting the prerequisites was not an easy task. I remember sitting on my screened porch in West Palm Beach after my first chemistry class, wondering what in the world I was getting myself into. I remember trying to come up with an attitude that would help me take on this task. Looking at the periodic chart of the elements, I remember thinking about how all of the scientific secrets of planet Earth were going to be revealed to me. Learning chemistry, physics, algebra, and geometry would give me an insight into understanding the Earth on a level I could have never imagined… But when I found out that I would have to dissect a cat in the anatomy class I was required to take, I almost changed my mind.

"I don't think I can cut up a cat," I said, fretting and complaining to my sister.

"If you think dissecting a cat is bad, it gets worse, because I think my chiropractor mentioned that he dissected cadavers."

I felt faint as I listened to the bad news. "Oh, no!" I cried. "That can't be true!"

My worst fears came true when I found out that, yes, I would have to spend one morning a week for two years in a cadaver lab. I dissected organs, muscles, tendons, ligaments as part of my training to learn how this magnificent body of ours works.

Looking back, I don't know how I did all that I had to do to become a chiropractor. Most people do not realize it, but course for course, the education of a chiropractor is very similar to that of a general practitioner medical doctor. The main difference is that medical doctors get a lot of training in using medications while chiropractors get a lot of training in learning about the relationship between the nervous system and the skeletal system. And chiropractors learn how to find and correct subluxations to release the miracle within.

Above, Down, Inside, Out

As a chiropractic student, I was introduced to the concept that health comes from **Above, Down, Inside, Out**—thus the **ADIO**, a word that would become a familiar abbreviation for what chiropractors believe to be true.

Healing is an innate power of the body that comes from above, down. The miracle within heals from the inside, out. Chiropractic adjustments remove interference to the miracle within.

There are all sorts of treatments and medications that can be tried to heal the body from the outside in. However, removing the interference to the vital force within and allowing the body to heal from the inside out is what chiropractic is all about. Healing comes from the miracle within, as demonstrated when a cut to the skin heals, leaving no trace of injury. The bandage removes the interference to healing, but the body heals itself.

This innate healing power of the body is transmitted to every cell through the nervous system. The nervous system is the body's communication system and the brain is the master computer of the body, which sends mental impulses down the spinal cord to control the function of every cell, tissue, and organ.

I like asking patients if they can guess which organ was the first organ that formed when they were in their mother's womb. They look at me with a puzzled look while thinking about the creation of their body. Most guess, "Was it the heart?"

Nope, it's not the heart. The brain is the first organ to emerge into physical form.

New Humans

When a sperm and egg unite, they become one cell. This cell then begins a process of division called mitosis. One becomes two, two becomes four, four becomes eight, and like compounded interest, the number of cells grow very quickly. Eighteen days after the fertilization of the egg, the brain can be recognized as the first organ of the body.

Then a tiny streak extends down from the brain. This "neural streak" becomes the spinal cord. The spinal cord is our lifeline, transmitting operating instructions from the brain to every cell of the body.

The nervous system, consisting of the brain, the spinal cord, and the nerves, is the first system of our body to emerge into the physical world. As the master computer of our body, the brain directs the creation of the body by sending mental impulses down the spinal cord and out through the nervous system to all parts of the body. At points along the spinal cord, organs begin to grow. After the brain, the second organ that can be recognized is the heart.

The twenty-six bones of your spinal column protect your spinal cord and give structural support to your body. There are cartilage disks between the bones providing a space for the spinal nerves to exit. The nerves are the communication system that the brain uses to deliver the operating instructions to every cell and organ of your body.

The spinal column and skeletal system are divided into four major sections:

- the head and neck
- the mid back
- the low back
- the pelvis and sacrum

The nerves exiting at various levels of the spinal column deliver mental impulses to the organs. For instance, the nerves exiting the neck are the nerve supply to structures such as the vocal cords. The nerves exiting the mid back include the nerve supply to the heart and lungs, and the nerves exiting the low back include the nerve supply to the intestines.

Subluxations impede the flow of mental impulses needed by the organs of the body to function properly. The innate intelligence of the body, connected to a Universal Intelligence, works through the brain to control every function of the body. Chiropractic adjustments release the miracle within by releasing the blockage to the innate intelligence of the body.

I will be giving specific examples of conditions related to subluxations in the different regions of the spine that show how chiropractic adjustments release the miracle within. A chart of the nervous system showing the relationship between the organs of the body and the bones of the spinal column is located at the end of this book.

The innate intelligence of the body created your body from two cells. All during your life, innate intelligence controls every function of the body. Our innate intelligence keeps our heart beating, our digestive system digesting, our lungs breathing, and other organs functioning throughout our entire life. Innate intelligence is the source of miracles within us, both large and small.

B.J. Palmer, known as the "developer" of chiropractic, wrote about innate intelligence in a very poetic way:

"We chiropractors work with the subtle substance of the soul. We release the imprisoned impulse, the tiny rivulet of force that emanates from the mind and flows over the nerves to the cells, and stirs them into life. We deal with the magic power that transforms common food into living, loving, thinking clay; that robes the earth with beauty, and hues and scents the flowers with the glory of the air."

When you suffer a physical injury, the innate intelligence of the body heals the injury. When you eat food, the innate intelligence of the body turns food into the living tissue of the body. Removing interference to the innate intelligence of your body allows for the natural healing of your body. All healing comes from within.

The miracle within is the innate intelligence of your body, which was responsible for the emergence of your physical body into the physical world.

Interference to Innate

There are three major types of stress that cause interference to the nervous system and lead to chiropractic problems: physical stress, chemical stress, and emotional stress.

Physical stress, such as a car crash or other trauma, overexercising, sleeping the wrong way, or a difficult birthing process can cause minor misalignments of the skeletal system that can be corrected by a chiropractic adjustment. Subluxations impede the flow of the vital life force. Chiropractic adjustments remove the interference to this flow.

Chemical stress, such as cigarette smoke, toxic fumes, or chemicals added to our food irritate the nervous system. As discussed, the mental impulses from the brain travel to every cell of the body via the nerves. But the opposite is also true. Our nervous system is a two-way street. Chemical stress is perceived by the nervous system, and the reaction to chemical stress can cause a subluxation.

And last but not least, emotional stress causes chemical and hormonal changes in the body, which irritate the nervous system and lead to subluxations.

Chapter Four
Subluxations—the Silent Killer

The title of this chapter may sound harsh, but it is true. Subluxations not only cause pain and discomfort, but they can lead to disease and death. They inhibit the flow of mental impulses from the brain that are necessary for the body to function at 100 percent. If a subluxation is preventing the vital energy from flowing easily to an organ, a subluxation can lead to a disease of that organ.

The word "subluxation" means "slight" (sub) and "dislocate" (luxate).

Correcting subluxations are what make chiropractors unique.

Subluxations are different from dislocations. A dislocation, such as a dislocated shoulder or finger, requires medical attention, whereas a subluxation requires the attention of a chiropractor. Many people are unaware of the dangers of a subluxation, but if maximum health potential is desired, subluxations must be found and corrected before damage to the body occurs.

There are five major components of a subluxation:

1) **The Bone Component** – Bones have a cartilage cap, and a subluxation causes the cartilage to become inflamed. A bone that is out of its proper position is not moving properly in relation to the bone above or below, causing stress on the ends of the bones. This mechanical stress on the ends of the bones causes the inflammation of the cartilage and begins the degenerative process known as arthritis. Neglecting to get a subluxation corrected can be compared to the wear and tear on your tires caused by driving a car that needs an alignment.

2) **The Nerve Component** – A subluxation impedes the flow of the vital energy needed by the body to function properly. If tissues and organs do not get the mental impulses they need, they begin to malfunction. These malfunctions manifest in various symptoms, depending upon where the subluxation is located. If a subluxation is located in the lumbar area, reducing the mental impulses to the intestines, disorders of the digestive system may develop. If the subluxation is located in the mid back, the nerves to the stomach, lungs, or liver cannot deliver the vital energy needed by these organs. Symptoms related to these organs can develop. If the subluxation is in the neck, symptoms related to the head, such as

headaches and stiff neck, can develop. Because every nerve in the body begins at the opening in the skull where the brain becomes the spinal cord, a subluxation in the neck can affect the entire body, causing symptoms from nervous tension to a case of the blahs.

3) **The Muscular Component** – Subluxations may cause irritations to the nerve supply to your muscles, causing aches, pains, and muscle spasms. Massage, physical therapy, and other modalities are helpful in treating the *symptoms* of a muscle spasm. But the *cause* of the spasm is a subluxation, which irritates the nerve supply to the muscle. A chiropractic adjustment corrects the *cause* of the muscle spasm.

4) **The Soft Tissue Component** – A subluxation also affects the surrounding soft tissue. Tendons, ligaments, and other tissues can become inflamed. If the subluxation is not corrected, permanent damage due to scar tissue formation and adhesions will leave the joint with a reduced range of motion. Chiropractic care maintains the mobility of the joints of the body. As the saying goes, "you are as young as your spine is flexible."

5) **The Chemical Component** – The body reacts to a subluxation by releasing chemical substances known as "kinans" that increase inflammation.

Over twenty years ago, before all the attention that inflammation is getting today, I had a professor who talked a lot about inflammation. He said it was not high cholesterol that was causing heart and artery problems, it was inflammation causing plaque buildup. As it turns out, he was right. Inflammation is a serious condition that is gaining more and more attention these days as being harmful to your health. Inflammation is being implicated in many different diseases.

Chapter Five
Believe It or Not

When it was discovered that the world was not flat, some people refused to believe it. They may have formed the "flat Earth society" in an attempt to hold on to their old way of thinking. Changing our minds about what we think to be true can be uncomfortable, but the good news is that changing what we believe to be true is possible. All we have to do is open our minds to new ideas.

The fact that you have an innate intelligence within you, which can bring forth healing miracles from within via a chiropractic adjustment, may still seem far-fetched to some. But as one wise old chiropractor once told me, "The truth always rises to the top."

You don't have to "believe" in chiropractic for it to work. Dr. Sid Williams, the founder of Life Chiropractic College, used to say, "It's like gravity, it works whether you believe it or not!" To illustrate his point, he would take his keys out of his pocket and drop them to the floor.

Dr. Sid had other favorite lines that he would share with his students during assembly.

- If you don't have a backbone, we can't help you.
- Try chiropractic first, medicine second, surgery last.
- Tell a chiropractor nothing; he will still get you well.
- There is one basic, underlying cause to most diseases.
- It's rare when a case doesn't respond to chiropractic.
- We promote chiropractic because we love mankind.
- We've seen people get well who've been sick for years.
- Chiropractic today for a healthy tomorrow.
- Those who shun chiropractic are probably sincerely ignorant on the matter.
- Medical treatment is welcome if that's what's needed.
- Chiropractic offers permanent relief in the shortest period of time at the lowest cost possible.
- You can be healthy and still need periodic adjustments for maintaining good health.
- The power that made the body is the same power that heals the body.
- Chiropractic works.

"I'll Give You One Shot"

I've had patients come in to my office and say, "I don't believe in chiropractic, but I'm going to give you one shot to see if this works."

If I determine that their problem is a chiropractic problem, I never hesitate to accept the challenge of a skeptical patient. As I tell these patients, you don't have to "believe" in chiropractic for it to work for you.

I've never had to "sell" chiropractic to my patients, because chiropractic sells itself. When a patient comes in for an adjustment and feels better after the adjustment, that's all I need to hear. The patients who give me "one shot" always call to give me "another shot," and eventually, many of the most skeptical patients become patients who realize the value of getting their subluxations corrected so that the vital energy of their body can flow more easily to keep their body in good working order.

I consider myself to be partners with my patients in their health care. If they want to come in for just one visit, that's fine with me. But I make sure they understand that sometimes, it takes more than one adjustment. It is true that sometimes it takes only one visit to get relief, but sometimes, it takes more.

You don't have to believe in chiropractic for it to work for you. But if you don't believe chiropractic will work for you, chances are, you won't even consider making an appointment to find out if what you are thinking is true.

Alyson's Miracle

Belief is a powerful force. I had a patient who illustrates this point. She was a patient who healed herself with her beliefs.

Take the case of Alyson, a young woman in her thirties. I tell her story to illustrate the fact that there is a healing miracle within us all, and we need to find out what it is that will release the miracle within us. For many people, it is the chiropractic adjustment that releases the miracle within. But for others, it may be something else.

Alyson had more nervous tension or stress than most patients. She worked at a newspaper, in the advertising department. She would come to see me once a week, and each time I saw her, I had to adjust the same subluxations over and over again. Although she would feel better for a day or two after her visit, she was not holding her adjustments, so she kept coming back to see me week after week.

I could see that she was under a lot of stress, and I made extra time to talk to her about ways to control it. I suggested counseling, yoga, deep-breathing exercises, reducing sugar and caffeine, and even taking a warm bath at night to help her relax. Nothing seemed to help. The best she could do was to get a weekly adjustment for some temporary relief.

Then one day, she came to see me, and I could tell there was a difference. She seemed more relaxed. In fact, she seemed quite relaxed, and she was anxious to tell me about the miracle within her.

She had gone to a church and talked to the pastor, and then attended the service on Easter Sunday.

"I looked at Jesus up on the cross and just turned all of my problems over to him," she said.

And obviously, she had done just that. I couldn't believe the change in her. I was amazed at the drastic change from one week to the next. She only needed a few adjustments that day. She made her usual appointment for the next week, and when she came back a week later, she had maintained her sense of serenity and she was holding her adjustments. Then she told me that she had decided to quit her job and go to work for the church. She found her miracle.

Chapter Six
Preventing Arthritis

We think of bone as a hard, rocklike substance, but in the body, bone is a living tissue that can change in accordance to the amount of stress placed upon it.

We have 206 bones in our skeletal system. (Interestingly, more than half the bones in our body are located in our hands and feet.) The junction where two bones meet is called a joint or an articulation.

The ends of bones are covered in a cartilage cap, which is lubricated by synovial fluid. In a healthy joint, the bones move smoothly against each other and life is good. But when subluxations increase stress on the joints, the cartilage becomes inflamed and the slow process known as degenerative joint disease begins. The process of degeneration of the ends of the bones that form joints is commonly known as arthritis.

"**Arth**" means joint and "**itis**" means inflammation. When two bones of the skeletal system are not moving properly in relation to each other due to the stress of a minor misalignment (a subluxation), it causes a fixation or the joint being "stuck." The joint becomes inflamed. If not corrected by a chiropractic adjustment, the cartilage that caps the ends of the bones begins to deteriorate. Degenerative joint disease is another word for arthritis.

Rick's Neck

One of my first patients came to see me complaining of pain in his neck that began after a strenuous day of working out at the gym. He was in his late sixties, and told me that he had been diagnosed with arthritis in his neck many years ago. Because of insurance requirements, I sent him out for an X-ray. Sure enough, I could see the degenerative signs of arthritis in his neck.

On an X-ray, bone appears white. The X-ray of a healthy spine shows a black space between the bones, representing a healthy cartilage disk.

We have a cartilage disk between each of the bones in our spinal column, which serve as spacers between the bones. A healthy cartilage disk is necessary so that the nerves extending out from between the bones can transmit the mental impulses to the body.

Showing Rick the X-ray taken from the side or lateral view of his neck, I pointed out how some of the disks were thinner than normal, especially the disk between the C5 and C6, located in the middle of his neck. His C5 disk was much thinner than the others. The disk was not doing a very good job acting as a spacer for the nerves or providing a cushion for the proper movement of C5 in relation to the bone above or the bone below. Bones are a living tissue and the bones in his neck had changed shape due to the stress placed on them. The bones of his cervical spine, which should normally look like square boxes with clean lines and spaces between them, were misshapen, especially C5, which had some "lipping and spurring," and other signs of degeneration due to the stress of the subluxation.

Continuing with my chiropractic exam, I found that C5 was the most subluxated vertebra in his cervical spine. It was rotated to the left and not properly articulating with C4 above it or with C6 below it. Ouch. No wonder he was in pain. Since he had never been to a chiropractor, I was quite certain that this problem was a long-standing predicament. He said that, yes, his neck had given him some pain and stiffness problems through the years, but usually, a week or two of pain medication had solved the problem. Or so he thought. His neck was decaying due to long-standing, uncorrected subluxations.

When it comes to many diseases, including arthritis, prevention is the best cure. Taking steps to avoid a problem is easier than trying to solve the problem once it happens. I do not tell patients that their problem could have been prevented had they known about chiropractic earlier in their life, because I do not want to make them feel bad. I do explain to them how periodic maintenance care can slow down the degeneration of their spinal column.

I explained to him that C5 is a common area of the cervical spine for arthritis, because C5 is the apex of the normal curve we have in our neck. This curve in our neck is designed by Innate Intelligence to give our neck the ability to balance our head on top, which is a pretty amazing feat since the head weighs more than ten pounds.

I explained to him what I found, what I was going to do, and how I was going to do it. I gently adjusted his spinal column where needed, including C5.

It took a few visits, but soon he was feeling better. He decided to become a maintenance patient. That is, he wanted to come in every five weeks to get checked in order to keep things in line.

I love adjusting maintenance patients. For me, a dream practice would be all maintenance patients! Maintenance patients are happy. They like feeling good. They understand the importance and value of getting their spinal columns checked for subluxations, and they take an active role in taking care of themselves. They live what I call "the chiropractic lifestyle." They pay attention to their health, and periodic chiropractic checkups keep the healing power of their bodies working at 100 percent of its potential.

Rick became a happy maintenance patient, but two years later, he injured himself again while working out at the gym. There was no traumatic impact and the pain did not begin until the next day, so I did not suspect any fracture. But he was interested in seeing another X-ray of his neck.

Lo and behold, we could both see that the miracle within him had been released—and the X-rays proved it. There was an amazing difference between the two lateral views of his cervical spine taken two years apart. There was less arthritis! The rough edges of the bones in his neck were less rough. There was more space between the bones. The amount of "lipping" and "spurring" had been decreased. The bones of his cervical spine looked better than two years prior.

"Look!" I said, looking at the X-rays of his neck as if I were looking at a photograph of him. "You look younger today than you did two years ago!"

"Can I get some wallet-sized photos for my Christmas cards?" he asked, feeling rather jovial while looking at the improvement that was visible on the X-rays.

Rick was amazed at the difference he could see in the X-rays of his neck. His neck *did* look younger in the new X-rays.

We talked about how most people think of bone as a hard, rocklike substance when, in reality, bone is a living tissue that changes in accordance to the stress upon it. Rick's chiropractic adjustments had reduced the stress on the bones, allowing the bones to remodel and release his miracle within.

He recovered quickly from this new sports injury and continued his maintenance care.

Sigh…

One day, many patients after that incident, I was browsing the magazine section of a large bookstore when an issue of *Newsweek* or *Time* magazine (cannot remember which) caught my eye. The cover story, in large letters, said, "Arthritis – The Coming Epidemic." The subtitle was something about the fact that baby boomers were getting older and, therefore, the number of people in our society who were going to suffer from this painful, debilitating disease was going to become an epidemic.

Filled with anticipation that I was about to read a story about the benefits of chiropractic care, I grabbed the magazine off the shelf. I sat down and flipped through the pages, looking for the story about how chiropractic care can prevent and help those afflicted with arthritis.

It was a long article, seventeen pages in all, with news about all the new drugs being developed that one could try. I kept turning the pages, thinking they were going to save the best news of all for last, but to my dismay, there was not one mention of chiropractic. I sighed a deep sigh of disappointment and put the magazine back on the rack. I promised myself that one day, I would write again to share much needed information and awareness about chiropractic that is lacking in most media outlets today.

The Limitation of Matter

It has been proven to me time and time again that the body has an amazing ability to heal. I believe where there is life, there is hope. There are miracles within us all, waiting to be released by chiropractic care. Sometimes, the joint is so far gone that the only alternative is surgery, assuming the patient is well enough to undergo the procedure.

I remember an elderly patient whose hip joints were so deteriorated that doctors said hip replacement surgery was out of the question. She used a walker and required assistance getting onto my adjusting table. It was a little bit too late to make any major improvement in her joints. She did get temporary relief from getting adjustments, which reduced the amount of nerve irritation. She was able to cut back on pain medication following an adjustment, so for her it was worth it. Unfortunately, hers was a case of "too little, too late."

The pelvis, which provides the foundation for the spinal column, has three parts: a left ilium, a right ilium, and a sacrum. The sacrum is a shield-shaped bone at the base of our spinal column. On either side of the sacrum are the left and right ilia. These are rounded bones that provide a shelf for mothers to carry their babies, for students to carry their books, or men to carry boxes. The left and right ilia also provide a place to put our hands when we feel the need to stand in defiance to look cool. One of the most important things about the left and right ilia is that they each have a socket for the hip joint.

It's My Sacroiliac!

The hip joint is a ball and socket joint. The ilium has the socket. The largest bone in the body, the femur, or thigh bone, has a ball at the end of it. An X-ray of a healthy pelvis shows that the hips joints have a nice space between the ball and socket, representing the cartilage cap of the ball and the cartilage lining of the socket.

A subluxation of the sacroiliac joint causes stress on the hip joint. This can lead to a wearing away of the cartilage and the degeneration of the hip joint.

The X-ray of the pelvis of the elderly patient who came into my office with a walker was shocking. Not only was the cartilage gone from both the ball of the femur and the socket of the ilium, but the femur had worked its way through the socket and was protruding into the ilium! *Good grief!* I thought to myself when she showed me her X-rays.

Because every nerve in the body begins in the neck, and because the degeneration of her hip joints was so severe, I decided that the best approach for this patient would be to check for subluxations in her neck. I explained that reducing the amount of nerve irritation in the upper cervical spine might give her some relief even in her lower body. Chiropractic care was not going to correct the cause of her problem, but it could help her feel more comfortable. She told me that whatever I could do to help ease her pain would be appreciated.

As it turned out, she did feel better with the upper cervical adjustments. She was able to reduce the amount of pain medication she was taking. She said that my adjustments were the best medicine for her pain. She was a sweet woman who was very appreciative of my care. I could not help but wonder what her life would have been like had she been under chiropractic care from a young age.

Chapter Seven
Chiropractic for Children

I did not get my first chiropractic adjustment until I was an adult, but looking back on my growing-up years, I know I could have used a chiropractic adjustment before that.

I remember that when I was in the eighth grade, my left arm would fall asleep. And when I turned my head a certain way, I would feel a rush of weird warmth running up the back of my head. Because my parents did not know about chiropractic, I was taken to a medical doctor and given some pills that made my face turn red. They lit me up like a Christmas tree. Looking back, what I needed was a chiropractic adjustment.

Children should be checked for subluxations. Many times, the first subluxation occurs during the birthing process. Twisting and pulling on the head while being born can be very traumatic, as I saw during a film at a Florida Chiropractic Society conference I attended in Orlando.

The video showed an actual birth. The person delivering the baby was pulling on the head and stretching the neck. The purpose of showing this video was to prove the presenter's point: the first subluxation oftentimes occurs at the moment of birth.

We do not hear about sudden infant death syndrome too much these days. When I was a chiropractic student, the standard of care for sleeping babies was to put them on their stomach with their head turned to one side. The theory we discussed was if the baby's head was turned to the side, a subluxation in the cervical spine increased stress on the brain stem. This situation could compromise vital functions, such as breathing and heartbeat, which are controlled by the brain stem.

Adjusting Babies

Many chiropractors adjust babies shortly after they are born. It only takes a light touch to gently align the upper cervical spine and give the baby a good chiropractic start to life.

I have adjusted babies with amazing results. One baby boy could not keep any food down. His parents brought him to the hospital and were told to try different formulas, but nothing was working. The grandmother was my patient and asked if I would take a look at him to see if I could detect any subluxations. I told her to tell his mother to put some shoes on him before bringing him in so I could get a good leg length check.

Performing a leg length check on a three-week-old baby to detect subluxations is done a little differently than for an adult. I gently laid the baby down face up on the adjusting table. Gently holding both feet, I let him draw his legs up to his chest and straighten them a few times, following their natural tendency to do so. Then, on the way down, I put the heels together and took a look to see that, yes, there was a short leg.

The only adjustment I do on babies is to adjust the very top bone in the neck. This bone, C1, is also known as atlas. It is the first bone under the opening in the skull where the brain becomes the spinal cord. A subluxation of C1 can cause all kinds of symptoms, including the fact that this baby could not hold down any food.

Using a very light pressure, I adjusted the baby's atlas. Within a few days, he was eating normally. On his next visit, his leg length check showed that he needed no further adjustments. His family was amazed and grateful that the baby's problem was solved. For me, it was just another miracle in the line of duty; a miracle within being released by a chiropractic adjustment.

As he grew up, he would accompany his mother and grandmother when they came in for their adjustments, and once in a while, he would want to get up on my table and have me check him. He delighted in getting up on my adjusting table. I always allowed him to have his turn, but I never found anything else to adjust.

Children love getting adjusted. I remember a little five-year-old boy whose parents understood the importance of getting their children checked by a chiropractor as part of getting a healthy start to life. After his first adjustment, he would come in with his parents and always wanted to be the first to get his adjustment, which both his parents and I found to be highly amusing.

One day, the mother of this little boy told him that she was going to come see me and get adjusted, and he said he didn't want to go. He was adamant, but because he was just five years old, he didn't have any choice, so she brought him in to my office. But he kept saying no, he didn't want to get onto the table. His mother convinced him to just get on the table and let me have a look, and lo and behold, his legs were perfectly even, and stayed even during all of the isolation reflex tests I performed. He knew he did not need an adjustment!

Scoliosis and the Little Cowgirl

Scoliosis is a condition of the spinal column that is characterized by an abnormal curvature. As a chiropractor, I was trained to detect and correct subluxations that may be associated with a scoliosis.

A quick screening test that can be done for children is to stand behind them, have them reach down as if to touch their toes, and then look at the "rib hump" of the back. Scoliosis appears as one side of their back rising up more than the other side.

A functional scoliosis is an abnormal curve caused by subluxations. Chiropractic care can improve or completely straighten a functional scoliosis if the patient has not yet reached the age of fifteen years. After the age of fifteen, the cartilage in the spinal column turns to bone and the scoliosis becomes permanent.

My first scoliosis patient was a shy seven-year-old little girl who came into my office wearing little cowboy boots. Her mother said they just found out she had scoliosis. A friend told her that she should bring her daughter in to get checked by a chiropractor to see if there was anything I could do to help her. Upon taking her case history, I learned that the only other health problem she had was wetting the bed.

The standard of care for "treating" scoliosis is to X-ray the child every six months to see if the curve worsens. When it reaches a certain point, a surgeon should be consulted to talk about bolting rods to the bones of the spinal column to straighten it out and prevent it from getting any worse.

Upon examination, I determined that the child did indeed have chiropractic subluxations of her pelvis, sacrum, and lumbar segments, especially L3, one of the bones in her lumbar spine.

Her mother watched as I went through the Activator Method protocol to find and correct her daughter's subluxations. Her leg length discrepancies were easy to see, and after I adjusted her, her leg lengths were even. When I saw how easy it was to figure out what needed to be adjusted and how balanced her legs became after the adjustment, I was very optimistic that she would get great results. I told her mother that I believed I found the basic, underlying cause of her problem, and her mother seemed hopeful.

I scheduled a follow up for later that week. I was surprised when her entire family showed up for the next appointment, including her grandparents. Her mother reported that she stopped wetting the bed the very same night of her first adjustment. The nerves that exit the spinal column at the level of L3 are the nerve supply to the bladder. The subluxation was reducing the mental impulses needed for the normal function of her bladder.

Upon examining her posture, we could see that her rib hump was totally within normal limits. Her miracle within was that there was no sign of scoliosis. There was nothing more to adjust. She was free from subluxations and free from a lifetime of suffering from scoliosis. The members of her family thanked me and shook my hand. It was a great experience for all of us.

I had another similar story with a thirteen-year-old girl who came in with X-rays showing moderate scoliosis. After a few adjustments, her mother said she was standing up straighter. Her mother wanted another X-ray, so one was ordered. Sure enough, the scoliosis had straightened out.

A Shortage of Chiropractors?

I hope that some of the children I have adjusted grow up to be chiropractors. As I tell many of my patients, someday there is probably going to be a shortage of chiropractors.

There are 316 million people living in the United States, seven billion people on the planet, and only about 60,000 chiropractors. If suddenly everyone woke up and realized that they should get their spine checked for subluxations, there would be lines of people down the street waiting to get into every chiropractor's office!

This statement, of course, raises eyebrows, but allows me to explain what I believe to be true.

Chiropractors are not spending billions of dollars every month to broadcast television commercials explaining the benefits of chiropractic care. People find out about chiropractic from other people, one spine at a time. Even though the chiropractic profession doesn't have the financial backing to spread the news about how chiropractic can improve health, the chiropractic profession is the fastest-growing segment of health care today.

The Tipping Point

There is a story, or perhaps a myth, about a phenomenon that was observed by scientists studying the behavior of monkeys. As the story goes, when a certain number of monkeys began washing their potatoes before eating them, monkeys on the other side of the world began washing their potatoes before eating them also.

This phenomenon is controversial among scientists as to whether or not it's true, but if it is true, there will come a time when droves of people suddenly realize how important it is to get their spine aligned. Then there would indeed be a shortage of chiropractors.

At the moment, the only humans who fully understand the value of chiropractic are chiropractors and educated chiropractic patients. My patients nod their head and agree with me when I pose questions, such as,

- Can you imagine how the health of our country would improve if everyone understood how important their brain and nervous system was to maintaining the health of their body?
- Can you imagine if there was a chiropractor in every doctor's office and that everyone who goes to see a health-care provider for whatever reason would get checked for subluxations?
- Can you imagine how good it would be if there was a chiropractor in every hospital and that everyone who goes to the hospital would get checked for subluxations?
- Can you imagine how the costs of providing health care to humanity would be reduced if the cause of the problem was corrected at the source before it became a disease?
- Can you imagine if every health-care professional agreed that the standard of care for

every human being is chiropractic first, drugs second, surgery last?

My patients like it when I talk like this. They nod their heads yes, and we stop for a moment to imagine the day when chiropractic care will be as commonplace as putting a Band-Aid® on a cut.

Chapter Eight
X-rays

Wilhelm Roentgen was a scientist who discovered X-rays quite "by chance" while conducting experiments of passing electric currents through a cathode ray tube. What he discovered was that the ray that was emitted from the other end of the tube was able to penetrate a nearby piece of cardboard that had some fluorescent crystals attached to it. He had never seen a ray like this before, so he called it an X-ray.

The first X-ray ever taken was of Roentgen's wife's hand. It was December 22, 1895. It took almost an hour of exposure to produce this first crude X-ray. A photo of this first X-ray in today's textbooks shows the picture of the bones in his wife's hand and the outline of her wedding band.

When Mrs. Roentgen saw this picture of the bones in her hand, she said, "I have seen my death." She was referring to the fact that the X-ray of her hand looked like a picture of a skeleton's hand.

I don't believe she was talking about her real death. I believe it was the image of her skeleton that inspired her comment. However, I was told in chiropractic college that Roentgen's experiments on his wife led to her early demise.

Thank goodness, major improvements have been made in the field of radiology. The film used in the process has a type of crystal coating that requires a much less powerful X-ray to get a good image, and lead shields are used to protect the body parts not being X-rayed. Today, X-rays are considered to be safe.

On an X-ray, bones appear to be white against black, and there is a lot of information that can be revealed from looking at an X-ray. X-rays show whether or not there is a fracture, a tumor, or any degenerative changes. X-rays also show many other things, too, such as abdominal aneurysms and signs of other serious problems.

Because it is difficult to see everything that can be seen on an X-ray, I send my patients to a radiologist to get X-rays. The radiologist reads the X-rays and writes a report that is delivered to my office, along with the X-rays, so that I can discuss the findings with my patient.

Sure, I can look at an X-ray and see arthritis, but there are things that I may miss, such as a tiny dot that may be the beginning of a cancerous tumor, an aneurysm of a major artery, signs of an infection, a disease process causing necrosis of bone tissue, or other pathologies that radiologists are trained to detect.

Although I choose to not take X-rays myself, I am grateful for the working relationship I have with radiologists, who provide me with detailed reports, describing what they find on the patients I send to them for X-rays. X-ray technology has come a long way and has become much safer than it was during the early days.

An X-ray shows a two-dimensional view of an anatomical structure and a CAT scan shows a three-dimensional view of a structure. However, a CAT scan also gives the patient more radiation. Studies have been performed to determine how dangerous X-rays can be, and physicians who X-ray their patients are required, by law, to tell the patient about the risks involved.

Did you know that in "the olden days," you could go into a shoe store, put on a pair of shoes, and step onto an X-ray machine to see how the bones of your feet looked in the shoes to make sure the fit was correct?

I found an online video of a film clip released by the United States Attorney General's office demonstrating what to look for in your feet when trying on a pair of shoes in a shoe store that had one of these newfangled X-ray machines.

I asked some of my older patients about these machines, and they remember them. "Yes!" said one, who recalled those days. "The picture of the bones in my feet looked green!"

Like many things, there is a risk-benefit ratio to be considered when making the decision to have an X-ray taken. In many cases, X-rays are required, but if not, careful consideration should be given to making that decision.

There are many chiropractors who would not dream of beginning chiropractic care without them, and some patients look forward to getting them. I am a chiropractor who does not order X-rays routinely in my practice. Because some people like X-rays and some do not, it is good to know that not all chiropractic techniques require X-rays.

Some chiropractic techniques require X-rays because some techniques involve measuring angles and widths. Those measurements are taken into consideration before determining the line of drive for the correction. Some chiropractors want to see the condition of the bones of the skeletal system before doing a manual manipulation. Some patients seem disappointed when I tell them I do not believe X-rays are necessary for their case.

Chiropractic care can be compared to what an orthodontist does, except without the braces! An orthodontist straightens the teeth and chiropractors straighten the bones of the skeletal system I am quite certain that an orthodontist would not dream of beginning orthodontic treatment without taking X-rays, just as there are chiropractors who would not dream of beginning chiropractic care without first taking X-rays.

As a chiropractic student, I was required to learn about several different chiropractic techniques before choosing which one was right for me. One particular technique, an upper cervical specific technique, involved taking X-rays of each other's necks. We then learned how to analyze the X-rays by drawing lines and taking measurements of the bones that could be seen on the X-ray.

The class required me to have two specific X-rays taken of my neck. One X-ray was taken through my open mouth to see C1 from the front to back, to determine if the number one vertebra under the opening in my skull had shifted to the left or right. Another X-ray was taken through the top of my head to determine if C1 had rotated.

This process of learning to take special X-rays, analyzing the X-rays, and determining how to adjust C1 took several weeks. I was looking forward to the big day when we would go into the clinic and use the upper cervical adjusting instrument to adjust each other.

In the process of learning to read the X-rays of my neck, I could see that my C1 was rotated posterior on the left. This could have happened during my birthing process, when I fell off my bike, or when I was hit from behind in an automobile accident. Regardless of how it happened, I could see for myself that the top bone in my neck was rotated out of its proper alignment with the opening in the base of my skull.

The night before my fellow students and I would finally be adjusting each other's atlas, I was walking down a grassy hill carrying my heavy book bag. It was a rainy night in Georgia, and Georgia mud is slippery when wet. The heavy book bag on one shoulder was throwing me off balance. Suddenly, my foot slipped out in front of me and I landed on my behind. I felt my head snap back. I had given myself a minor whiplash.

I got up, shook it off, and kept walking, pretending to myself that it never happened. The next day, I felt soreness in my upper back and shoulders, but did not say anything. As many people might do, I ignored the fact that I may have suffered a subluxation of my neck.

I was taught that an episode such as this could definitely change the measurements of the atlas that were needed to set the dials on the upper cervical adjusting instrument that we were learning to use. I knew that the upper cervical technique might require new X-rays to determine new settings for the adjusting instrument, but I was a student who didn't want to delay the process of fulfilling my class assignment.

The atlas adjustment is an important adjustment. The proper alignment of atlas, in relation to the opening in the bottom of the skull where the brain becomes the spinal cord, allows the flow of mental impulses from the brain to bring healing energy to every cell of the body.

Dr. Sid, the president of Life Chiropractic College, told us students that he believed the upper cervical subluxation was responsible for many problems affecting humans. He believed that subluxations of one's atlas, besides causing physical problems, can cause unclear thinking. As an extreme example, to illustrate his point, he told us that he believed prisons and hospitals were filled with people who have a major subluxation of their atlas.

Because X-ray analysis showed my C1 needed to be adjusted on the left, my student clinician instructed me to lie on the adjusting table with my left side up. After making sure I was in the right position, she set the dials on the instrument according to the analysis she did of my upper cervical spine *before my fall on the Georgia mud.* Placing the stylus over my C1, just behind my ear, she pressed the lever that moved the stylus and adjusted my atlas.

Afterward, everyone in the class was talking about how good they felt after getting their C1 adjusted. But not me. I did not feel so good. By the next day, I had an abnormal sensation going down my left arm. My imagination began working overtime as I found myself wondering if I might be having a heart attack.

When I told my professor what happened, she sent me to the college research department, where the top upper cervical chiropractors in the country were doing research.

Like my original injury suffered in my automobile accident, this minor whiplash suffered by falling on my behind in the Georgia mud was another blessing in disguise. I was now under the care of the top upper cervical doctors in the world.

New X-rays were taken of my upper cervical spine. Even though I am one of those people who does not prefer X-rays unless absolutely necessary, I am very grateful for the technology.

After my C1 was adjusted properly, I went back to my biochemistry class and sat in the back of the room so as not to disturb anyone by my late arrival. I felt good. My arm no longer hurt. My mind felt clear. Amazingly, I felt as if I could see more clearly! I felt that I could breathe better! I was experiencing what thousands of my patients now experience. The power had been turned on. The vital life force was flowing from above, down, and out to every part of my body. I was feeling the miracle within.

Chapter Nine
Cervical Spine (the Neck)

We have seven bones in our neck, C1 through C7. The letter C refers to the fact that the anatomical name of the neck is the cervical spine. Subluxations in the neck can lead to symptoms such as headaches, dizziness, and high blood pressure.

C1 – Atlas

The very first bone just beneath the opening in the skull where the brain becomes the spinal cord is C1, also known as atlas. C1 was named after Atlas, the mythological character who holds planet Earth on his head.

Illustrations of Atlas show him as a big, strong fellow doing an amazing job of holding the world above his shoulders. It seems like an impossible job for one man, but for a mythological creature such as Atlas, balancing the weight of the world on his shoulders is no problem.

Chiropractors named the top bone in our neck after Atlas, because our atlas plays an important role in maintaining the balance between our neck and our head. The atlas is a ring of bone that weighs about an ounce. The human head weighs between ten and twelve pounds.

Some chiropractors believe that the atlas is the most important bone in the body due to its proximity to the brain stem and the fact that the nerve supply to every cell in the body can be traced back to the level of C1.

Every nerve in the body begins at the base of the skull, and injuries to the atlas can result in devastation.

Christopher Reeves

Christopher Reeves suffered fractures of both C1 and C2 in a horse jumping accident that left him paralyzed and unable to breathe on his own. He needed a ventilator because his body lost the ability to inhale air into his lungs.

Exhaling does not require effort, but inhaling air into the body requires mental impulses from the brain being sent to the muscles that control breathing. The brain sends mental impulses to the diaphragm, intercostal and neck muscles to maintain normal breathing. In the case of Reeves, the injury to C1 and C2 interfered with the communication from the brain to the respiratory muscles, making it impossible for him to breathe on his own. However, he did make progress with respiratory therapy exercises, and at one point, he was able to breathe for thirty minutes without the use of a ventilator.

His tragic accident illustrates the importance of the vertebrae in the upper cervical spine.

Adjusting Atlas

While I was a student at Life Chiropractic College, I studied with Dr. Roy Sweat, an upper cervical doctor in Atlanta who developed the "Atlas Orthogonal" technique. I worked in his office one day a week and was amazed to see that both patients and medical doctors came from all over the world to see him.

One day, while sitting at the X-ray view table, learning how to analyze the line of correction for C1 from a set of cervical X-rays, there was a group of medical doctors who came all the way from Japan to his Atlanta office to specifically learn about adjusting C1. They were a friendly group who took a lot of pictures.

There was a German medical doctor who brought his wife from Germany to see Dr. Sweat after she had a stroke. Pictures of her face taken before and after the adjustment of atlas were amazing. Her drooping eye and face were completely back to normal. The improvement in her appearance began within minutes of her adjustment, demonstrating the miracle within.

I appreciate everything I learned from the renowned Dr. Sweat about adjusting the C1 vertebra, but because I am a chiropractor who prefers not to use X-rays, I chose the Activator Method instead. As it is often said at chiropractic conferences, and as I said earlier, "it's not the technique, it's the technician."

All the many different chiropractic techniques work. It is a matter of personal preference for the chiropractic students to learn the technique that feels best for them. Ultimately, that is a good thing. People are different and every individual has a preference as to what type of health care they receive.

Bell's Palsy

I have had successes similar to what I saw in Dr. Sweat's office by adjusting atlas using the Activator Method. Two amazing cases come to mind.

A fifty-five-year-old woman was referred to me by her massage therapist. She was diagnosed with Bell's palsy, and was told nothing could be done for her. She came into my office with one side of her face drooping. She had never been to a chiropractor before. She was upset, unhappy, and desperate to find a solution to her problem.

Using the Activator Method analysis, it was easy for me to see what segments of her cervical spine needed to be adjusted. As she lay face down on the table, I asked to perform the isolation test for C5, which is lifting her face off the table. This isolation test of C5 increased the stress on C5 and one leg pulled short, a reflex that let me see quite easily that C5 needed to be adjusted. In a similar way, having her tuck her chin increased stress on C1, I found her atlas was also subluxated. Using my Activator adjusting instrument, I made the adjustments and saw that her legs became balanced. This objective observation told me that a major correction had been made to her neck.

The next day, she came into my office looking like a different person. I almost did not recognize her. Not only was her face not drooping, but she was smiling. She told me how she was amazed at what happened after her chiropractic adjustment. She could not believe how much better her face was. She told me that her neighbors and family sat around the table with her last evening, "watching her face come back!" She was thankful that she gave chiropractic a chance to release the miracle within.

With teary eyes, she opened a bag and presented me with a little statue of an angel, which I added to my collection of angels that have been given to me by my grateful patients. These angels inspire me, make me smile, and remind me of the miracle within.

Extreme Dizziness

Another story of an amazing result with adjusting C1 was of a man who was brought to my office for extreme dizziness. He was under the care of a medical doctor at Mayo Clinic in Scottsdale, who prescribed drugs for dizziness. But the patient was not getting any better. It took him several minutes to stand up from the chair in the waiting room and make his way into my adjusting room.

As I proceeded to examine the patient for chiropractic subluxations, I could not believe how short his leg got in second position, that is, when I lifted his legs to take a look at the leg length discrepancy. There was a four-inch difference! I began my analysis and found that not only was C1 subluxated, but C2 and the back of his skull were also subluxated. I adjusted all three segments, mentioning to him that having three major subluxations in a row was putting an enormous amount of pressure on his brain stem at the top of his spinal cord.

He took a few breaths and began walking around my office. He sat down in the chair and stood up much more quickly than before, looking at me with wonder in his eyes. The friend who brought him in to see me was the first to speak.

"Is it better?"

We both looked at the patient, waiting for him to reply. He looked at me and then looked at his friend, and sat down. When he stood up again, he whispered, "I think so."

I was surprised that he was so subdued about it. Maybe he did not really believe how such a little tap to his neck could make such a huge difference.

He told me he had an appointment with his doctor at Mayo the next day, but scheduled an appointment for the day after that.

When he came in for his follow up, he was feeling much better. He had less dizziness and was able to stand up from a seated position quite readily.

"I told my doctor at Mayo what you did and he wrote it down on my chart," he said, as if this was the most unusual thing about his chiropractic experience.

I remember thinking after he left that I should drive over to the Mayo Clinic and offer my services one day a week. I never did, but I see a future where someday, medical doctors and chiropractors can work together to do what is best for the patient. Having chiropractors on the staff of all hospitals to check patients for subluxations could go a long way in improving our current system of health care.

Like many, this patient became a maintenance patient and referred many patients to me. He understood the importance of maintaining a proper alignment of the bones in the spinal column.

Dehydration Dizziness

I had another case of a patient with dizziness who did not respond to my adjustments. Surprisingly, I was not able to help her. It was a patient I saw weeks before for low back pain, and she was now coming to see me complaining of dizziness.

I found and corrected her cervical subluxations, and told her to come back the next day. When she came back, she was no better. I checked her and found that she needed another adjustment, and told her to come back again the next day. Again, she was no better and still complained of dizziness. I thought maybe she had an inner infection, a sinus infection, or some other medical condition, so I told her that she should go see her medical doctor as soon as possible to get a diagnosis.

The next time I saw her, she was fine. She told me her medical doctor took one look at the palm of her hand and could see from the shriveled skin on her fingers that she was severely dehydrated.

"I drive in my car all day for work and I do not drink much water because I do not want to have to stop and use the restroom. I got myself dehydrated," she explained.

I took a deep breath. You learn something every day. Now, when a patient complains of dizziness, the first thing I ask them is if they have been drinking enough water.

C1 – Headaches

A subluxation of C1 is a common cause of headaches.

C5 – the "Stress Vertebra"

The anatomy of a healthy neck includes a gentle curve, which provides a biomechanical advantage to support our head. Many cervical bed pillows are designed to support this cervical curve. The C5 vertebra is located in the middle of our neck, at the apex of our cervical curve. As the apex of the cervical curve, C5 is under a lot of stress, thus the nickname of "stress vertebra." Arthritis in the neck usually begins with C5.

C5 is the nerve supply to the vocal cords. When I was practicing in Nashville, several of my patients in the music business made their living by singing. These singing patients appreciated that I checked their C5 to make sure that the power to their vocal cords was operating at 100 percent peak efficiency. A dimmer switch to the vocal cords is not something any singer would want.

C7 – Nerve Supply to the Thyroid Gland

There are seven cervical vertebrae. C7 is located at the base of the neck, where the upper back begins, and is the nerve supply to the thyroid gland.

C7 has the nickname "vertebral prominens," because it is so prominent. If you reach around and touch the skin at the base of your neck, you will feel C7 "sticking out." Most people never notice their vertebral prominens until they have a pain that seems to be coming from that area. I have had patients who become concerned when they discover it.

"Doc, something's wrong there. Feel it. It feels like a bump sticking out." I reassure them it is not abnormal. We all have that feature.

Maintaining a healthy cervical spine is important in maintaining the health of the entire body. I recommend head and neck exercises for maintaining a healthy neck. As an added benefit, this exercise helps the brain and eyesight because it drains waste products from the head.

Draining Waste from the Brain

The brain uses more energy than any other organ in your body. This energy is created through biochemical processes in the body, which turns the food you eat into fuel for your brain.

Food becomes energy for the muscles and organs through a biochemical process called the Krebs cycle. The Krebs cycle is a series of chemical reactions that occur in the mitochondria of every cell in our body. As in many chemical reactions, there are waste products that must be eliminated by the body. These waste products are leftover pieces of molecules called metabolites.

Because the brain uses more energy than any other organ in the body and has more Krebs cycle activity than any other organ, the brain creates a large amount of metabolites that need to be eliminated from the tissues of the brain.

Antioxidants

One of the most popular metabolites that nearly everyone knows about is an atom of oxygen. At the end of a Krebs cycle, a single atom of oxygen is left over. This lonely atom of oxygen has a chemical tendency to connect to other atoms. The problem with this tendency is that a single atom of oxygen causes oxidation. That is, whatever it attaches to begins to oxidize or rust. These single atoms of oxygen can destroy cell walls and cause damage to the body.

Antioxidants scoop up the atom of oxygen and make it less harmful to the body. Fruits and vegetables have a lot of antioxidants, which make them good choices for your diet.

Head and Neck Exercises

Alzheimer's disease has been shown to possibly be a buildup of plaque in the brain. I wonder if plaque might be caused by accumulated metabolites that were not drained from the brain.

Researchers say that what is good for the heart is good for the brain. They also suggest that exercise may help prevent Alzheimer's disease because it increases blood flow to the brain. I wonder if an exercise that removes metabolites from the brain can help prevent Alzheimer's...

The lymph system can be compared to the circulatory system, except the lymph system does not have a heart to pump the lymph through the lymph vessels. Lymph depends on the muscular movement of the body to do its job.

The lymph system is part of the sewage system of our blood. Blood flows through the lymph nodes, which filter waste. The lymph system collects the waste from the blood and eliminates it through the digestive system.

Because of the amount of waste products produced by the brain, we have a large concentration of lymph nodes at the base of the skull and in the neck, which help filter the blood from the brain. The head and neck exercises assist this cleaning process by draining the brain and stimulating the lymph nodes, which filter the blood.

It is a common recommendation to check with your doctor before beginning any new exercise program. This is very good advice. As a chiropractor, I highly recommend you also check with your chiropractor to make sure you don't have any chiropractic problems with the bones in your neck before beginning these head and neck exercises.

1) The first head and neck exercise is to bend the head forward toward the chest, slowly and carefully. Do this three times. Hold it there for a moment as you feel the muscles relax. Doing this slowly, and with your full attention to the activity, also give the neck and shoulder muscles a nice stretch. Breathing deeply and slowly while doing these exercises releases tension in the muscles, tendons, and ligaments.

2) Now gently tilt the head to the back three times, very slowly, while shrugging the shoulders. *I always recommend shrugging the shoulders while tilting the head back.* Shrugging the shoulders toward the ears, while tilting the head back, protects the neck. It also compresses the lymph nodes at the base of the head, squeezing the waste products out of the lymph nodes and sending it on its way to the thoracic duct for proper disposal into the intestines.

To help my patients remember this exercise, I tell them they can combine the head and neck exercises with some positive affirmations. When nodding their head, they can say, "Yes, today is going to be a good day."

3) The next exercise is to turn the head from side to side, very slowly, as if saying no. "No negative thoughts or negative people are going to interfere with me having a good day." Do this three times.

4) Now, tilt the head over to one shoulder, three times, very slowly. Then tilt the head toward the opposite shoulder, three times, and then straighten. I call this movement "maybe." "Maybe something really good will happen today!"

5) When the neck has been stretched and warmed up with these beneficial stretches, the final exercise is to do head rolls, *remembering to shrug the shoulders when going back.* Roll the head slowly three times in one direction, then reverse the process by rolling the head three times the other way.

These head and neck exercises are a good way to start the day and end the day. They can be done sitting on the side of the bed.

Chapter Ten
Thoracic Spine T1 – T12
(the Mid Back)

Beneath the seven bones in our neck are twelve bones of the thoracic spine. These twelve vertebrae are unique. They have ribs attached to them. The ribs extend around to the front of our body, forming the rib cage, which is designed to give support to our body and protect our lungs.

T1 – Nerve Supply to the Lower Arms and Hands

T1, the first of twelve thoracic vertebrae, is located just beneath C7, the last bone in the neck. The nerves that exit the spinal column at the level of T1 travel down the arms and into the hands.

A chiropractic subluxation of T1 can produce symptoms of carpal tunnel syndrome. Sometimes, nerve interference is not coming from the hand, but from higher up. More about the carpal tunnel will be discussed in the section on extremities. If the problem in the carpal tunnel is due to a subluxation of T1, this will be revealed during a chiropractic exam. When a patient complains of symptoms in their hands and elbows, I always check T1.

T2-T3 – The Nerve Supply to the Heart and Lungs

"Don't forget to check my T2 and my T3," says one of my patients who comes in every month or two for a spinal "tune up" and adjustment.

He had open heart surgery and wants to be sure that the nerve supply to his heart is turned on to full capacity.

I am not treating his heart. He is under the care of a cardiologist who repaired his heart and saved his life. I remove the interference to the nerve impulses that go from his brain to his heart.

The heart beats constantly from the moment we are born until the moment of our death. Correcting chiropractic subluxations at the level of T2 ensures that the heart is getting mental impulses it needs from the brain to function at 100 percent of its potential.

Technically, he comes to see me for his low back pain. When the bone in his back, known as L4, gets misaligned, he feels a pain in the right side of his low back. When L4 is subluxated, his foot catches when he walks and he almost trips, a condition known as "foot drop." The cause of his foot drop is the lack of nerve supply to the foot, which can be traced to his lumbar spine.

"I can tell how badly out of alignment L4 is when not only does my low back ache, but my right foot does not lift the way it should when I am walking on the treadmill. I find myself struggling to keep my feet moving properly," he says, "but don't forget to check T2 and T3 also."

I love it when patients are involved in their care and understand what I do.

Chest Pains

One of my patients went to the emergency room because he was having chest pains. He came to see me on the way home from the hospital. I was glad he went there first because that is where I would have sent him had he come into my office first!

A series of tests at the hospital showed no signs of heart problems. The emergency room doctor told him that it might just be stress. He left the hospital and called me to get checked for subluxations. This is an example of a chiropractic patient who understood the importance of being checked for subluxations no matter what the symptom might be.

I found that two ribs needed to be adjusted on the front of his rib cage, just over his heart. He was not sure what he did to cause such a subluxation, but I have seen it several times in my practice. Anterior rib subluxations can cause symptoms that mimic heart problems.

My vision is that someday, everyone will consider the possibility of nerve interference for all health problems.

The Lungs

T2 and T3 are also the exit points in the spinal column for the nerves supply to the lungs. A reduced amount of vital force flowing from the brain through the openings between T2 and T3 is a dimmer switch that reduces the mental impulses needed by the lungs to function at 100 percent of their health potential.

When the nerve supply to the lungs is compromised due to a subluxation of T2 and T3, the lungs can become susceptible to diseases, including asthma, emphysema, and chronic obstructive pulmonary disease.

I remember a mother who brought her little boy in to get his adjustment when his asthma would flare up. She said he could breathe easier by the time he got home, and his adjustment seemed to make his medication even more effective.

T4 – Nerve Supply to the Gallbladder

The gallbladder is a pear-shaped organ tucked beneath the liver on the right side of our body, under the last rib and beneath the right breast. During an exam of the abdomen, doctors will reach up under that rib to see if they can feel the liver. Hopefully, they won't. If they do, it means that the liver has begun to harden. This happens in diseases of the liver, including cirrhosis.

The liver produces bile, which is then stored in the gallbladder. Bile is a nasty-smelling liquid that emulsifies and helps digest fat. When we eat fat, the gallbladder squirts bile into the digestive tract to help break it down.

About 750,000 people a year have their gallbladders surgically removed because they are inflamed and full of sludge and gallstones.

I had the opportunity to watch a video of the procedure one Thanksgiving Day, when a family member brought the souvenir video of his surgery to the gathering. He asked if anyone wanted to watch it. As a chiropractic student, I was the only one interested in watching it with him.

Removing the gallbladder is a laparoscopic procedure. By cutting a few holes into the upper abdomen, a camera and some tools designed for the procedure can be inserted to easily do the job.

Soon thereafter, I had another opportunity to see the gallbladder. This time it was up close and personal - during cadaver dissection lab. The students in the lab were divided into four teams. We each had our own cadaver that we would visit once a week.

One day, when we were all dissecting the thoracic cavity of our particular cadaver, a team on the other side of the lab was abuzz about something they found inside their cadaver.

I left my cadaver and walked over to see what the commotion was all about. What in the world was this? It resembled a green balloon stretched out over the liver. We came to the conclusion that it was most likely a burst gallbladder.

The gallbladder is not a spare part, but people can lead normal lives without one. The body has an amazing ability to adapt. After a gallbladder is removed, the liver sends a constant trickle of bile into the digestive tract.

T4 is the nerve supply to the gallbladder. When the gallbladder becomes diseased, the pain sometimes radiates into the upper right side of the back. I have had patients with pain in the upper right quadrant of their body. They think it might be a chiropractic problem, but sometimes it is a symptom of a gallbladder that is beyond repair.

If an adjustment does not lessen the pain, I refer them to their medical doctor for an evaluation. A simple ultrasound exam will reveal if there is a problem with the gallbladder, such as gallstones or sludge. Sometimes, a gallstone can become lodged in one of the ducts. This can be a very serious problem that requires immediate medical attention.

A fully functioning body requires a flow of impulses from the brain to every cell and organ. I have seen many patients with subluxations that could be impeding the nerve supply to their organs. Long-standing subluxations of the spinal column can reduce the nerve supply to the associated organ, which can lead to the disease of the organ.

Interestingly, because the gallbladder stores bile, which is produced in the liver, some health professionals believe that gallbladder problems begin in the liver. If the liver is not functioning properly, the quality of bile may not be good. Bad bile could lead to sludge and gallstones in the gallbladder.

T5-T6 – Nerve Supply to the Stomach and the Liver

T5 and T6 are the nerve supply to the liver and the stomach. When these are subluxated, symptoms related to stomach and liver conditions may result. This is not to say that everyone with subluxations of certain levels will develop conditions related to these organs. However, an occasional chiropractic checkup to make sure the "power is turned on" is a good preventative maintenance to ensure your organs are receiving the nerve supply they need to stay healthy.

Most people go to see a chiropractor for neck and back pain because that is the niche that chiropractors have carved for themselves in the world of health care. Preventative maintenance is to ensure that the signals from the brain that travel down the spinal column reach every cell and organ of the body. Chiropractic maintenance care is a low-cost insurance policy that will pay great dividends in the long-term health of the human body.

T7 – Diabetes and the Pancreas

T7 is the nerve supply to the pancreas. The pancreas makes insulin, which controls blood sugar levels. If the pancreas is not working properly, problems with blood sugar could arise, including diabetes.

The American Diabetes Association reported that in 2011, a total of eighteen point eight million children and adults living in the United States have been diagnosed with diabetes.

When I was a chiropractic student, I was taught that there is no such thing as "prediabetes." Either your pancreas is working properly or it is not. Since then, a new classification has been adopted that puts "prediabetes" into a separate category from diabetes. The American Diabetes Association states that seventy-nine million people have prediabetes.

According to the Centers for Disease Control, diabetes is the seventh leading cause of death in the United States. The possible complications from the disease include heart disease, stroke, blindness, kidney disease, neuropathy, and amputation.

The cost of diabetes, updated March 6, 2013 by the American Diabetes Association, is $245 billion. That figure includes $176 billion for medical costs and $69 billion in reduced productivity.

The cells of the pancreas are supposed to secrete insulin to keep the blood sugar at a healthy level. Everyone should know if their pancreas is working properly or not. Anyone can go to the pharmacy and purchase a kit for testing blood sugar. A device that holds a tiny lance which automatically pricks the finger. A testing strip inserted into the meter gives your blood sugar level. A prescription is not needed to purchase this and it is a good idea for everyone to monitor their blood sugar level.

It is also a good idea to make sure there are no subluxations interfering with the nerve supply to the pancreas. Regular chiropractic checkups and adjustments are good preventative measures to ensure that the pancreas is getting all the mental impulses it needs to function at 100 percent of its potential.

Some diabetics have to inject themselves with insulin. Nowadays, they have an insulin pump that attaches to a permanent port for delivering predetermined amounts of insulin into their abdomen. Diabetics find this to be more convenient than having to inject their abdomen several times a day. However, testing the blood sugar throughout the day still requires pricking the finger. Some diabetics are able to take an oral medication to keep their blood sugar level.

Diabetes

I received a phone call from a former patient who wanted to share good news about her daughter, who was diagnosed with Type II diabetes one year ago.

At the time of her daughter's diagnosis, the mother was very upset that her child had to go through having to learn and manage Type II diabetes. She was horrified that her daughter would have to wear a permanent insulin pump and monitor her blood sugar level by pricking her finger several times a day.

My patient understood that chiropractic care improves the nerve flow to the organs of the body, so she brought her daughter in to see me. The young woman had no aches or pains. Her problem was diabetes.

I explained to her that the nerves that exit the level of T7 are the nerves to the pancreas, and if there is a subluxation at that level, the power to the pancreas would be diminished.

The results of my chiropractic exam showed me that her daughter needed several adjustments, including T7. After four visits, the only subluxation still showing was T7. I was able to adjust her T7 on several more visits until she moved away.

The good news that her mother wanted to report was that somehow, her daughter's pancreas had begun working again. She was happy to report that although the doctors could not explain why, they were able to remove the pump. Her daughter was now able to manage her blood sugar levels by taking medication.

"Her father and I are convinced that getting her T7 adjusted helped her pancreas."

My vision is that every patient who seeks medical attention will be checked for subluxations as part of every routine health exam. Getting checked for chiropractic subluxations to make sure the power that made your body is flowing easily to every cell and organ of your body is one of the best things you can do for your health.

T8 – The Immune System

T8, located at the bra line, is the nerve supply to the spleen. The spleen, located on the left side under the ribs, is part of our immune system. It makes some of the white blood cells that fight bacteria. An adjustment to T8 turns on the power to the immune system and helps keep us healthy.

I teach my patients that if they feel their resistance is low, the first thing to do is to find out if T8 needs to be adjusted. When a subluxation of T8 gets adjusted, the power to the immune system is restored.

T9 – The Adrenal Glands

T9 is the nerve supply to the adrenal glands. The adrenal glands produce stress hormones such as adrenalin and cortisol. The adrenal glands are part of the "fight or flight" system of our body. This feature was helpful in the days when primitive humans came face-to-face with a wild animal. A decision had to be made. Were they going to stay and fight or take flight?

Either way, the situation called for the adrenal glands to squirt adrenalin into the bloodstream. The adrenalin rush causes changes to the nervous system that give us the burst of energy needed in emergency situations. Blood from the digestive system is sent to the muscles, slowing down digestion and preparing the muscles for quick action. Whether staying to fight the tiger or run for our life, the body is prepared to take massive action.

This ancient fight or flight mechanism is still working within us today, but rather than a tiger or wild animal, the stress we face is the stress of everyday life. The constant stream of chemicals released into our bloodstream irritates the nervous system and cause subluxations.

Learning to manage stress is an important part of keeping ourselves healthy. More about this will be discussed in a later chapter. In the meantime, take a couple of deep breaths and relax…☺

T10 – Nerve Supply to the Kidneys

I am happy to be on a mission of sharing my patient success stories with others, to show that chiropractic is important for releasing the healing miracle within.

To prepare myself for this new phase of my life of telling others what I know to be true about the healing of the human body, I attended a Toastmasters meeting and listened to a woman give a speech (of all things!) about her "Mysterious Medical Miracle."

She told the story of how, one day, she woke up feeling extremely tired. Dragging herself to the shower, she wondered why in the world she was feeling so badly. Halfway through the shower, feeling even worse, she turned the water off, got out of the shower, and sat down. She called her mother, and asked her to come over and take her to the clinic.

When she got to the clinic, they did some blood work and told her to get to the emergency room because something was terribly wrong. Before passing out, she was told that her kidneys had stopped working.

Much to her dismay, she was ordered by her medical doctor to have dialysis three times a week. She told the Toastmasters that she chose to have dialysis on Mondays, Wednesdays, and Fridays so that she would have her weekends free. She also mentioned that the needle used for dialysis was very large and the process was very uncomfortable.

Accepting her fate, she did her best to get back to living her life as normally as possible. One day, while driving her car, she was hit from behind in a car crash. She was transported to the hospital and admitted for observation.

The next day, her doctor came in to see her and said that there was something about her blood work that was puzzling. Her kidney function seemed to be improved.

"You mean I can skip dialysis?" she asked hopefully.

"No, let's wait and test this again tomorrow," he said cautiously.

The next day, blood tests showed the same thing— improved kidney function.

I sat there quietly, listening and thinking, and wondering if anyone was thinking the same thing I was thinking. I knew that was highly unlikely. I probably would have seemed strange to many of those attending, especially since the meeting was being held in the community room of a hospital. There are not too many chiropractors in hospitals yet, although I hope someday, that will change.

She ended her talk by showing us the beautiful afghan she knitted during her time spent in dialysis, and everyone clapped when she finished her story. Her story had a very happy ending. Because of her mysterious miracle, her kidneys were working again and she was able to stop dialysis. It was a miracle that no one could explain.

I found myself deep in thought. T10 is the root of the nerve supply to the kidneys. A subluxation at the level of T10 could have been the cause of her kidneys shutting down. Perhaps the jolt of the accident released the fixation of that part of her thoracic spine and released the miracle within.

At the end of the meeting, they asked if I would like to say a few words. I stood up and introduced myself as a chiropractor. I sat down without sharing what I thought about this mysterious miracle. Driving home, I thought to myself that chiropractors do not speak up enough to tell the world what we know about how the body heals itself.

I know the brain is the master computer of the body. Every function of every organ depends on the mental impulses from the brain to work at 100 percent peak efficiency. The brain and nervous system control every function of the body, including the kidneys. If the nerve supply to the kidneys is shut down by a subluxation, the kidneys will not get the mental impulses they need to function properly.

This particular Toastmasters club meets twice a month, and I received an e-mail inviting me back again. I plan to go back, join the club, and begin giving talks about what I know concerning the nerve supply to the organs of the body.

T12 – Nerve Supply to the Fallopian Tubes

Infertility

While taking the case history of a patient who came to see me for low back pain, I learned that she and her husband had been trying to get pregnant for almost two years. Upon my examination, I found that she had several subluxations, including her T12 vertebra. I explained to her that the nerve supply to her fallopian tubes exited her spinal column at the level of T12. I told her that from what I found during my examination, there was a possibility that there was nerve interference to her fallopian tubes. She was more than happy and willing to get that subluxation adjusted.

I am always happy to find subluxations that correspond with the patient's complaints because, oftentimes, their subluxation is the basic, underlying cause of their problem.

Several weeks later, she came in and was elated to tell me that she was pregnant. She said she and her husband were so excited and so happy. She was convinced that her subluxation of T12 was preventing her from getting pregnant. I am certainly not a fertility doctor; however, making sure that the nerve supply to the fallopian tubes is functioning at 100 percent of its potential is certainly a factor. It could not hurt.

Soon thereafter, she brought her husband, who wanted to meet me and was curious to see what I do. He happened to be a medical doctor. I was happy to explain to him what I do and how chiropractic adjustments affect the body. I told him that I believe everyone, as part of a wellness exam, should be checked for subluxations in order to remove interference to the nervous system.

After meeting me and listening to my explanation of what chiropractors do, he wanted me to check him for subluxations. He was not complaining about neck or back pain, but understood that chiropractors do more than just treat pain. He agreed that what I do is beneficial for the health of the entire body.

I adjusted the new mother during her pregnancy. I corrected subluxations of her pelvis and lumbar spine as they developed, and not surprising to me, she had a pain-free pregnancy and an easy delivery. The baby was completely normal and needed no chiropractic adjustment.

Besides being the nerve supply to the Fallopian tubes, T12 is a transition vertebra. T12 is the last vertebra in the thoracic spine and your last rib is attached to T12. When turning the trunk of the body, as when swinging a golf club, T12 gets a lot of torque. Those who play tennis and golf often have a subluxation at the level of T12, which can cause back pain.

The Golfer Guy

When I was practicing in Arizona, my sister was the headliner pianist at the Phoenician Resort in Scottsdale. She called me one day to say she met a golfer who had flown to Scottsdale for a week of golf, but he hurt his back and could not play. She said he had never been to a chiropractor, but she knew I could help him. She told him about me and wanted to know if I would be willing to bring my portable table to the Phoenician and adjust him. He was in tremendous pain and could hardly walk.

I agreed to go. I loaded my portable table into my car and drove to the Phoenician Resort, where I found a very unhappy golfer in a lot of pain. He said the pain came on suddenly while he was swinging the golf club. He tried to continue playing, but the pain made him stop. This was his golfing vacation and he was very unhappy about this "revolting development."

I set my table up and did my chiropractic exam. I found that he had a subluxation of L4 and T12. He was very easy to analyze. After I adjusted him, I knew he was going to feel much better. I told him to use ice for ten minutes each hour and to call me if he felt he needed another adjustment. I figured he would be well enough to drive to my office if he needed a follow up.

Later that day, he was in the lobby of the Phoenician, telling everyone about his miracle within. The adjustment had removed the interference to the nerve and he was feeling great relief. He told my sister that he thought I had "special powers." The truth of the matter is that the chiropractic adjustment has special powers. It can release the miracle within.

Many golfers understand the benefits of chiropractic care and get adjusted regularly to keep them at the top of their game, including Tiger Woods, who said, "I've been going to a chiropractor as long as I can remember. It is as important to my training as the practice of my swing."

Case closed.

Chapter Eleven
Lumbar Spine (the Low Back)

As the premise of this book states, chiropractors are more than just doctors for neck and back pain. The chiropractic adjustment turns on the healing power of the body, not just to the muscles, but to every organ of the body. Some of the most dramatic miracles I see in my practice are in adjusting the lumbar spine, not just for back pain, but for problems with the large intestine.

L2 – Nerve Supply to the Large Intestine

Problems with the large intestine range from constipation, colitis, irritable bowel syndrome, Crohn's disease, dysentery, diarrhea, appendicitis, cramps, and whatever else you can think of that would be related to "tummy troubles."

Perhaps the most dramatic miracles I see in my practice are related to the nerve supply to the large intestine.

When a patient told me that her fourteen-year-old daughter was suffering from Crohn's disease, I got out my chart of the nervous system and explained to the mother that perhaps the nerve supply to her daughter's intestines was being reduced by a subluxation in her lumbar spine.

Like many people, when I first went to a chiropractor for my own neck and back pain, I thought chiropractors were neck and back doctors. Little did I know that pain was just the tip of the iceberg. Chiropractic care improves the health of the entire body by removing interference to the nerves of every cell and organ of the body.

From my experience of seeing chiropractic adjustments turn on the healing power to the organs of the body, it sounded to me as if the nerve supply to her daughter's intestines was being compromised by subluxations. I was intrigued as to what I would find during my chiropractic exam.

I never adjusted a patient with Crohn's disease before, but the name of the disease did not matter to me. As a chiropractor, I do not name the disease, nor do I treat the disease. I correct the cause of the disease, no matter what organ is involved. Correcting the subluxation removes the interference to the nerves and allows the innate intelligence of the body to heal itself.

The Garden Hose Analogy

The brain controls every bodily function. The brain is the master computer of the body, and sends out mental impulses that are the operating instructions for every organ of the body. The nerves are the communication system from the brain to every organ and cell of the body. These power lines need to be kept clear of interference.

I like using the garden hose analogy to explain this concept to my patients. If you step on a garden hose, the water cannot get through. And if you cannot water your garden, the plants will wither and die.

A subluxation of the spinal column can be explained in a similar manner. If the mental impulses from the brain cannot get through to the organs because of a minor misalignment of the spinal segment, the organs will wither and die. A degenerative condition of an organ can be looked at as a withered organ.

If the intestines are not receiving the mental impulses through the nervous system, which they need to function properly, the result could be a disease with a name, such as Crohn's disease. My mission as a chiropractor is to find and correct the areas of the spinal column that are preventing the life force from flowing through the body, and thwarting the miracle within to be released.

When I saw my patient's daughter with Crohn's disease, I took her case history. I performed my chiropractic exam, which included her lying facedown my table and examining her legs to see if there was nerve irritation, causing one leg to pull short. There was. One leg was more than one inch shorter than the other.

When I lifted her legs up to take a look at how the leg lengths changed, in what we call the second position, her leg pulled about three inches short. I asked her to put her left arm across her low back, which is a test that increases the stress on the lumbar spine. Her leg pulled three inches short.

Her mother gasped. "Oh my God," she said. "Look at that!"

"It's okay," I said, remaining calm and finding something positive to say about this situation, which looked as if she was in desperate need of a chiropractic adjustment. "This is good," I announced. "It is going to be easy to see what is out of alignment."

After adjusting the subluxations in her spinal column, her legs balanced out.

"That is unbelievable!" her mother exclaimed, seeing that her daughter's legs balanced out after the adjustment. The mother had never seen that before because every time she came in to get her adjustment, she was facedown and could not see how her own leg lengths changed in accordance with what needed to be adjusted.

I told my patient and her mother that she might be a little sore after the adjustment because toxins would be released as the deep muscles surrounding her spinal column relaxed and lactic acid was discharged from the muscles.

When a muscle contracts, a chemical reaction takes place and lactic acid is produced. When there is a subluxation, the muscles of the body are in a constant state of contraction. I tell my patients that these tight muscles are like "lactic acid factories." Because the muscle is in a state of contraction, the blood cannot flow freely to the muscle, which is necessary to flush the lactic acid out of the muscle. A subluxation causes the muscles to produce and store lactic acid.

We have over three hundred muscles in our body. Many of them are tiny muscles that are attached to the bones of our spinal column. When unable to relax due to the nerve interference caused by a subluxation, these muscles become like lactic acid factories, producing more and more lactic acid that cannot be released due to the muscle tension.

A chiropractic adjustment reduces the amount of nerve interference and allows the muscle to relax. When the muscle relaxes, lactic acid is released into the bloodstream. Discharging lactic acid from tight muscles may cause soreness following an adjustment.

I always suggest that patients drink extra water after an adjustment to help flush out the lactic acid that may be released when tight muscles begin to relax.

After scheduling a follow-up visit, they left my office.

In her case, the amount of toxins and lactic acid released from the muscles of her body and intestines resulted in her feeling very ill after her first adjustment. She spent the next two days in bed, missing school one day and feeling awful, but they trusted the chiropractic process. By the time she came back for her next appointment, she was feeling much better and was ready for another adjustment.

On the second visit, my objective observation showed a significant improvement in her leg length tests, and she never again experienced any soreness from getting an adjustment. Within weeks, as her symptoms improved, her doctors were able to significantly reduce the amount of medication she needed.

Chiropractic care is a powerful healing technique that can help relieve the suffering of people, no matter what the health problem may be. Yet sometimes, it seems that chiropractic is the best-kept secret in the world.

L3 – Nerve Supply to the Knee

I like finding and adjusting L3 on patients who have pain in their knees. Removing interference to the nerves that go from the low back segment of L3 can make the knees feel better! Most people would never consider that a chiropractic subluxation of L3 could cause knee problems. Most times, when people have pain in their knees, they think there is something wrong with the knee.

I had a patient who came to see me several years after his knee replacement. He complained that low back pain prevented him from working in his yard. Upon taking his case history, I learned about his knee replacement surgery a few years prior, and I asked how his knee was doing.

"The doctor messed it up," he said. "I have pain all along the side of my knee since the surgery, but the doctor could not find anything wrong with it. According to him, the knee surgery went fine, but I think he messed up."

During my chiropractic exam, I found the usual suspects in his low back: a subluxated sacrum and lumbar vertebrae. Of special interest to me was L3, the nerve supply to the knee. This patient had a subluxation of L3. I adjusted it, along with the other segments that needed to be adjusted.

When he came back for his follow up, he reported that his low back was feeling much better. I asked him about his knee.

"It's better, too."

These are the miracles that chiropractors take for granted. These are the miracles "in the line of duty" that happen every day in every chiropractic office in the world. These are the miracles that will someday make chiropractors the saving grace of health care.

There are some knee problems that are too far gone. When the cartilage wears away due to long-standing subluxations, the only solution is to replace the knee joint with an artificial one. Chiropractic care prior to the surgery can improve the outcome and recovery time, as I have seen in my patients who needed knee replacements.

Pending Joint Replacements

Some patients choose to see their medical doctors in conjunction with their chiropractic visits. They understand that they need both. I fully support their decision. I work with them to help them prepare for the surgery by finding and correcting their subluxations prior to the surgery.

I have had amazing experiences adjusting patients who needed hip and knee replacements. No, I did not fix the joint so they did not need surgery; there is a limitation to matter and a limitation to what chiropractic can do. Perhaps if I had been adjusting them their whole life, they would not need a joint replacement, but that is another story.

One patient who needed a knee replacement got adjusted once a week right up until the week of his knee surgery. Two weeks later, he came walking into my office without a walker. He was smiling and very proud, and happy that he was doing so well.

"My doctor cannot believe it," he said.

"Did you tell him that you got adjusted right up until the time of your surgery?" I asked.

"No, I did not mention it to him," he replied sheepishly.

Looking back on those cases, I wish I could have discussed their cases with their surgeons, but many patients do not want their doctors to know that they are seeing a chiropractor. I have referred many patients to orthopedic surgeons when needed. Chiropractors working in conjunction with medical doctors will make the patient's outcome better. I look forward to the day when all health-care professionals work together for the highest good of their patients.

L4 – Sciatica

As previously discussed, L4 is the nerve supply to the muscles of the low back and to the prostate gland. It is also one of the roots of the sciatic nerve, a large nerve that extends from the lumbar spine down to the leg.

The spinal cord can be likened to a coaxial cable. A cross section of the spinal cord shows many different "cables" making up the cord. The spinal cord ends at the level of L2. The "cables" then branch out, forming an anatomical structure called the "caudal equine," which means "horse's tail" because that is what it looks like.

In chiropractic college, after two quarters of removing all the organs from the body and dissecting them, and two quarters of dissecting all of the muscles and tendons to see which bones they attach to, we finally got to the good stuff: the brain and spinal cord. (As a side note, walking across the cadaver lab with a lung in my gloved hands, I was amazed at how light it was.)

Besides the gloves, I wore two layers of face masks and a special set of clothes and shoes, which I kept separate and laundered separately for the special days in cadaver lab. Looking back, I do not know how I got through that portion of my training, but when one is on a mission, it is easy to ignore those things that are outside one's comfort zone.

Anatomy books say the sciatic is the largest nerve in the body, but to me, the spinal cord looked like the biggest nerve. It extends down from the brain and ends in the middle of the low back at the level of L2. The spinal cord then branches out, continuing as thick strands of nerves that travel through the spinal column and exit from the lower lumbar vertebrae. These nerves form the nerve supply to the lower body, including the legs.

The large nerves that exit from between L3, L4, and L5 are the roots of the sciatic nerve, a frequent cause of thigh and leg pain when there is a subluxation of the lumbar vertebrae. The sciatic nerve is about the thickness of your little finger. A subluxation of one of the lumbar vertebrae puts pressure on this nerve and causes the pain that is commonly referred to as "sciatica."

There is more to L4 than just sciatica. The nerves that exit L4 are also the nerve supply to the prostate gland.

L4 – The Prostate Gland

I had a young man who came to see me for low back pain. Upon taking his case history, I found that he was being treated for an inflamed prostate gland. His prostate symptoms included difficulty with urination.

A subluxation of his lumbar vertebrae can be compared to a dimmer switch that is turned down low, reducing the amount of mental impulses from his brain to his low back and his prostate gland.

Upon examination, I found that he had a subluxation at L4. Not only was his subluxation reducing the nerve supply to the muscles of his low back, but it was cutting down on the amount of the vital power needed by his prostate gland.

"Side Effects"

After two or three visits, not only did his low back feel much better, but he noticed an improvement in his prostate symptoms, a "side effect" of the miracle within. He was under the care of a medical doctor. As stated previously, as a chiropractor, I do not treat prostate problems or any other kind of disease process. I *do* find and correct minor misalignments of the spinal column, which allow the natural, innate healing energy of the body to do the healing from above, down, inside, and out.

I explained to my patient and he understood that keeping L4 adjusted was beneficial to his prostate gland. Even after his low back felt better, he came in for maintenance visits because his prostate symptoms were less with chiropractic care.

He was on medication for his prostate condition, and once again, he was another patient who was convinced that the chiropractic care he was receiving was making his medications more effective.

Articular Fixations – The "Miracle Cure"

As a chiropractic student, I remember a professor at Life Chiropractic College telling us that "articular fixations are the miracles." An articular fixation happens when a bone suddenly goes out of alignment due to trauma, such as moving a piano or lifting something heavy while twisting or turning. These articular fixations, when adjusted, return to normal relatively quickly, and seem like miracles.

My first articular fixation patient showed up when I was in practice for about six months. One of my patients called to ask if she could bring in her boyfriend because he hurt his back moving a piano. When she told me how much pain he was having, I suggested to his girlfriend that she may want to take him to the emergency room. Usually, people in that much pain call 911.

She said he did not want to go to the emergency room. He knew how much I helped his girlfriend, so he wanted to try chiropractic first. He did not want to be given pain pills and muscle relaxers. I scheduled his appointment.

I was a little flabbergasted when he showed up with two friends who had to practically carry him into my office. He was in an enormous amount of pain.

I figured I had one shot. If we could get him on my table facedown, I could take a look at his leg lengths, see which one is short, do a reflex isolation test, pressure test to figure out which bone was causing the pressure on the nerves, and using the handheld, spring-loaded instrument, I could adjust him. If that did not help, I would strongly suggest that he go to the emergency room.

Thankfully, I was able to lower the table to knee height. His friends were able to help get him on the table. He was moaning and yelling. I was perspiring. (Ladies do not sweat.)

When I was a chiropractic student, a professor told us never to use exclamatory words when examining a patient. Never say, "Oh my God, this is really bad!" Nor were we supposed to gasp. So I took a few deep breaths, kept my cool, and began my analysis.

His right leg was pulled two inches short, an effect of the nerve irritation to the root of his sciatic nerve. No wonder he was moaning in pain. When I lifted his legs an inch off the table, I could see that the right leg became even shorter. This told me it was L4, rotated posterior on the left, and pinching the root of the spinal nerve on the right.

I took my Activator adjusting instrument in one hand, palpated his lumbar spine, placed the Activator adjusting instrument to the left side of L4, and made the adjustment. Then I checked his pelvis and neck, did a few more adjustments, and I was done.

"That's it? That's all you're going to do?" he and his entourage asked incredulously.

"Yup, that's it," I said. I saw that his right leg was now level with the left and knew that I reduced the pressure on the root of his sciatic nerve.

His friends helped him get off the table. He stood up with a quizzical look on his face. "I think it feels better," he said softly. His friends stood there looking at him, and then at me, with wide eyes. For a long moment, the room was silent.

"Good," I said. "Go home and put ice on it for ten minutes at the top of the hour and five minutes at the bottom of the hour for as many times as you can tonight, and I'll see you tomorrow."

I called him a couple of hours later to see how he was doing. His girlfriend said he was resting comfortably and was feeling much better. If he had not been better, I would have suggested she take him to the emergency room for an evaluation. My feeling and philosophy are to try chiropractic first and see how that goes. Lucky for this fellow, he saw how chiropractic helped his girlfriend, and he decided to try chiropractic first. To his amazement and to the amazement of his friends, it worked for him.

Sometimes, the cartilage disk between the bones gets torn away from the bone. When a piece of the disk breaks away and lodges against the nerve, surgery is often necessary. MRIs and X-rays help diagnose these conditions. Since what I do is noninvasive, and if I believe chiropractic adjustments will help, I say chiropractic first.

If a patient does not respond in a few visits, or if there has been an accident and I suspect there might be a fracture, I immediately send patients to a medical facility for evaluation and X-rays. If an adjustment or two helps the patient, it makes the patient, their family, and me very happy.

I will never forget the look on his face when he showed up at my office the next day. He was smiling.

"I'm better! Much better!" he said. "I cannot believe it. What did you do with that thing?" he asked, pointing to my Activator adjusting instrument.

I explained to him again how I found and corrected the subluxation of L4 in his low back.

"It's unbelievable," he kept saying. "I can't believe one little tap with that thing could make such a difference. I can't believe how much better I feel. I know how much you helped my girlfriend, but I still can't believe how much better I am."

"Better is my favorite word in the English language!" I said, as I often do when patients tell me they are better.

I checked him again and found that a minor adjustment was needed to the sacrum at the base of his spine and another small adjustment was needed to L4. I scheduled one more visit with him. He called the day of the appointment to tell me that he was completely better and he did not think he needed to come in. I explained that there still might be some corrective work to be done and that we cannot always go by symptoms to determine if there is a subluxation. He was happy with the way he was feeling and told me he would call me if he ever needed me again.

I never saw him again, although his girlfriend continued coming in for maintenance treatments. When I asked about him, she said he was doing fine and was still talking about his experience with chiropractic care.

Making a House Call

A young man in his twenties called and asked if I could adjust people with rods in their backs. I told him I could. He told me more about his condition, and I realized that his case was probably beyond help. But since he heard me say I could adjust patients with rods in their backs, he would not take "no" for an answer. When he told me he was in a wheelchair, I offered to make a house call.

When I arrived at his home, I was met by his loving wife, who looked at me imploringly. The young man was sitting in a wheelchair in the living room. He told me how painful the rods were at the base of his spine, and was anxious to find out if there was anything I could do to help him.

Off to the side was a hospital bed with a pulley system they used to get him in and out of bed. I knew that he was suffering from what I call the "limitation of matter." There is only so much healing that a body can achieve. There are limits to what can be done. I knew he was beyond getting relief from a chiropractic adjustment. I thought about adjusting his cervical spine and some chiropractors may have done so. When I palpated his neck, my innate intelligence told me to stay away.

I was a chiropractor for a very short time and didn't have much experience in this type of situation. I was wondering what to say or do. He looked at me with suffering eyes. "I want to sit at my desk and get back to work, but I can't sit up without these rods causing pain in my low back."

Pain Is an Emotion

Even though I do not do physical therapy treatments in my office, I had to become certified in physical therapy to practice chiropractic in both Florida and Arizona. The physical therapist who taught the course said that pain is really an emotion because it is interpreted in our brain through the limbic system, which is the system that perceives emotions.

He was under the care of medical doctors. He had a mental health counselor, support from his church and family, but there was nothing I could do to help him. I told him I was sorry, but before I left, I gave him a suggestion.

The reality was that without the rods, he would not be able to sit up at all. I suggested if he could change his perception of the rods, he may be able to reduce his feelings of pain. Instead of hating the rods, he could be grateful that they, at least, allow him to sit up in a wheelchair. He looked at me thoughtfully and nodded his head yes, as if he understood.

When I got back into my car, I hoped my suggestion would make a difference in his life.

Chapter Twelve
The Pelvis and Sacrum

The sacrum has a big job to do. Located at the base of the spinal column, the entire weight of the upper body rests upon the sacrum, which is located in the center of the pelvis. If you have a subluxation of the sacrum, it hurts when you stand up from a seated position.

Robert the Architect

Robert is an architect who showed up in my office in an extreme amount of pain. He was leaning to one side and could not stand up straight. I had him do a couple of orthopedic screening tests to see if it was perhaps a herniated disk, but those tests were negative.

When he told me that it hurt the most when he stood up after sitting in a chair, I knew before he even got on my table that it was probably a subluxation of his sacrum. It was. His sacrum had somehow moved out of its proper position and was exerting pressure on the nerves. Following the adjustment, he felt immediate relief, and by the next day, he was completely better. His was one of those "easy to analyze, easy to fix" cases of the miracle within.

Robert was an interesting case, because the only adjustment he needed was an adjustment of the sacrum. About a month later, he showed up at my office again in a lot of pain, and once again, his subluxated sacrum responded to the chiropractic adjustment.

When it happened the third time, I knew there was something amiss. I asked him some detailed questions about his living and working activities. I asked him if he could think of anything he was doing that might be putting stress on his sacroiliac joints. I was looking for an answer related to ergonomics and body mechanics.

He realized that several times during his workday, he was bending over and reaching into a file cabinet next to his drafting table. Bingo! That was the answer. His improper stretching and reaching was causing the subluxation. He took immediate action. He changed the location of his office files, and became yet another sacrum success story who referred several patients to me.

The Body Adapts to Subluxations

The body has an amazing ability to adapt to the subluxation. When one segment of the spinal column or pelvis goes out of alignment, another segment usually compensates. Compensations are the body's attempt to adapt to a subluxation. Compensation is usually thought of as a payment for something, but to a chiropractor, compensation is when one subluxation leads to another.

Sometimes, everything that needs to be adjusted is found during my initial exam. Every so often, only the compensations will show up on the first visit, which is why I encourage patients to schedule a follow-up visit.

Compensations are a common reason why, in some cases, back pain goes away on its own. Perhaps the pain is gone, but the skeletal system compensates for the subluxation by creating another subluxation, as the story of my patient, Lori, illustrates.

Lori's Lateral Sacrum

Lori was a new patient complaining of low back pain that radiated to the right side of her low back. Like many low back patients, she was "easy to analyze and easy to correct." Her legs immediately balanced after the adjustment, and as she got off the table, I could see that the miracle within her had been released.

She had a surprised and grateful look on her face. She was nodding her head yes and smiling. "It feels better," she said.

The only subluxation I could find in her low back was L4. There was no sign of a subluxation in her pelvis or sacrum. I told her that might mean her pelvis and sacrum were fine. Or...the lumbar spine might be compensating for a subluxation of the pelvis. I explained that undoing compensations is sometimes like "peeling the layers of an onion," allowing the underlying subluxations to show up.

I had her stand up, walk around, sit down, and stand up a few times. Then I checked her again.

"Nope, no sacrum or pelvis adjustment needed. Just L4," I said.

I explained to her that if indeed L4 was compensating, it may take a few adjustments to "peel away" the compensations before the pelvis or sacrum would show up.

This was her first chiropractic adjustment ever. She had been in pain for almost a month. Because of the long duration of the pain, I had a feeling that her body was perhaps compensating to adapt to the original subluxation. This is a compelling reason to get to your chiropractor at the first sign of any pain or discomfort.

"If the sacrum or pelvis is released and needs to be adjusted, then the pain might come back and feel as if it's lower in your back," I warned her. She understood and promised to call me if she needed me.

Less than thirty minutes later, she called me. "My back is really hurting," she said. "Now the pain is lower in my back."

I told her to come back to my office and made way for her in my busy schedule, knowing that another miracle was about to be released from within.

Sure enough, when she lay down on my adjusting table, I could see that there was a leg length difference. But this time, it was the sacrum, the shield-shaped bone at the end of the spine that needed to be adjusted. It moved to the left and L4 had been compensating for it, just as I had suspected. After adjusting L4, the body was able to release the sacrum, and it needed to be adjusted. I explained to her that this usually only happens one time. Once my patients know about chiropractic, they come in to get the subluxation corrected as soon as they can, before it causes other subluxations.

I checked the left and right ilium that articulate with the sacrum and make up the pelvis, but there was nothing more to be adjusted. I had her get up from the table, walk around, sit down, and stand up a few times.

"It's better," she said, nodding her head yes and taking a deep sigh of relief. "I'm so glad you explained this to me. I had no idea what to expect. You made it easy for me to understand how this all works."

We scheduled a follow up. I gave her instructions to call me if she was anything other than better, because I might have to adjust her sooner than her next scheduled appointment.

I sometimes wonder if people who say that they only went to a chiropractor once and never went back were not educated on this important concept. Getting one adjustment might take care of the compensation subluxation. Afterward, when the basic, underlying subluxation causing the problem shows up, patients may experience discomfort and decide to cancel their follow-up appointment. These patients may be the ones who tell their friends that the chiropractor "hurt them."

Chapter Thirteen
The Extremities

The extremities are the parts of the skeletal system other than the spinal column. This includes the hands, feet, shoulders, and jaw. Many chiropractic techniques, including the Activator Method, address the subluxations that can occur in the extremities.

TMJ – Jaw Pain

The mandible, or jaw bone, is attached to our skull at a place known as the temporal bone. When we have trouble in our temporal mandibular joint, we call it "TMJ."

One day, while shopping at a health food store, I noticed a woman who kept putting her hand on her cheek. She was working behind the counter, and I could tell that she was in pain. I thought perhaps she had a toothache. When it was my turn to check out, I asked her what was wrong. She told me that she was having a problem with her jaw. She said that she was going to have to have surgery soon to fix it, and that her jaw was going to be wired closed for six weeks. She looked desperate.

I told her I was a chiropractor. I invited her to come to my office so I could examine her to determine if she might have a chiropractic problem. I gave her my card and she called to schedule an appointment. Sure enough, using the Activator Method protocol, I found that there was a subluxation of her temporal mandibular joint.

Using an extremely light setting on the Activator adjusting instrument and placing my thumb between the instrument and her jaw, I adjusted her TMJ and voila! The pain was gone!

She cancelled her surgery and was grateful that her jaw was not going to be wired shut for six weeks. Her problem was solved with one adjustment. I had a steady stream of new patients from her store for many years after that.

The Carpal Tunnel

One of my favorite childhood songs says, "The arm bone's connected to the hand bone," but what the song doesn't say is that between the arm bone and the hand bone are the wrist bones. There are eight bones in each wrist, which help form an anatomical structure called the carpal tunnel. Formed by bands of connective tissue in the wrist, the carpal tunnel is a passageway through which the nerves from the neck get to the hands.

When something goes wrong with the carpal tunnel, we call it carpal tunnel syndrome. Symptoms of carpal tunnel syndrome include pain, tingling, and numbness in the hand, arm, and wrist.

The nerves to the hands can be traced back to the neck. Many times, carpal tunnel symptoms are caused by a subluxation in the neck.

Sometimes, the subluxation causing carpal tunnel syndrome is located in the wrist. Either way, carpal tunnel syndrome is oftentimes caused by a subluxation that can be corrected with a chiropractic adjustment.

One of the bones of the wrist is called the lunate because it is shaped like a quarter moon. Because the lunate bone is located next to the carpal tunnel, a subluxation of the lunate can cause interference to the nerve that goes through the carpal tunnel. When nerve interference is affecting the transmission of the mental impulses from the brain to the hand, we get carpal tunnel syndrome.

Sometimes, carpal tunnel surgery is needed to clear the pathway of the carpal tunnel, but chiropractic subluxations of the wrist or neck should also be considered.

Ted the Tennis Player

Ted was unable to raise his elbow above his shoulder for years. He had never been to a chiropractor, but he missed playing tennis so much that he decided to give it a try.

As it turned out, he had a subluxation that was quite easy to find and correct. Immediately upon getting up from the table, he could raise his arm over his head. He was so happy that I do not think he heard me when I told him to take it easy and give his body a chance to heal. I think the only thing he was thinking about was getting back onto the tennis court.

Two days later, he came back to my office. He was in more pain than the first time I saw him. He told me that he felt so much better after that first adjustment. He was so excited that he was able to lift his arm normally again that he went out and played tennis for several hours. Because he did not take my advice to take it easy and give it a chance to heal, he suffered a setback from doing too much too soon following an adjustment.

It took several weeks before he was well enough to play tennis again, but he learned his lesson and took it slowly. He used ice for short periods of time after playing, and only played twice a week to allow his body to recuperate.

I am happy to report that he went back to playing tennis on a regular basis. Once again able to fully engage in one of his life's passions, he has become an enthusiastic advocate of chiropractic, and referred many of his fellow tennis players to me.

The Body Needs Time to Heal

Seeing patients engage in too much activity after getting relief from an adjustment, and then injuring themselves again, made it necessary for me to explain to patients that it takes time for the body to heal. I make sure they understand that even though they are feeling better, they should not go out and do all the things they have not been able to do.

When the pressure on the nerve is reduced by a chiropractic adjustment, patients often feel better immediately. However, the surrounding soft tissues of the body, including the muscles, tendons, and ligaments, need time to recover from the subluxation.

I explain that just because the symptoms have gone away, it does not mean that the body is fully healed. To illustrate the point that symptoms are not always a good indicator of whether or not there is a health problem, I ask the question, "What is the most common first symptom of heart problems?"

After pondering the answer to my question, I tell them that the most common first symptom of heart problems is death. They are flabbergasted to hear this, but it is true. Many people do not realize they have a heart problem until they have a heart attack and die.

My point is that we cannot always go by symptoms. This also goes for thinking that because the pain has subsided after a chiropractic adjustment, you are completely healed. The body needs time to heal and to acclimate to the new alignment following a chiropractic adjustment.

Maintaining Mike's Machine

I had a patient who was a college student and star pitcher for the college baseball team. Nothing was really hurting him. He had some stiffness and soreness across his shoulders, symptoms most people would call "normal."

His parents, living in another state, were seeing an Activator doctor there and wanted their son to get checked for subluxations. They found me on the Activator.com Website and told him to call me to make an appointment. He took his parents' advice and made an appointment.

Sure enough, his right scapula was slightly out of alignment. Using the Activator Method protocol, I adjusted his shoulder and arm. He became a regular patient. Not only did the stiffness in his shoulders and upper back go away, but he said the team had a device for measuring the speed of his pitch. After getting his adjustment, the speed of his pitch increased. When the speed of his pitch slowed down, he knew it was time to come get adjusted again. Another miracle in the line of duty.

Childbirth and the Tailbone

I got a call from my gynecologist one day, asking me if she could send over a patient who was having severe tailbone pain after childbirth. The mother could not even sit down to nurse her baby. She was exhausted, and was missing out on the joy of motherhood.

Upon examination, I found that, yes the coccyx had subluxated during the delivery and needed to be adjusted. I adjusted her coccyx and her pain began to subside. The mother was so grateful.

On another occasion, the same gynecologist called me, saying that she had another patient who was really in pain. "I think I may have broken her tailbone during the delivery. It was a tough one."

I told her that she needed to send her for an X-ray, because fractured bones are beyond the scope of chiropractic. As it turned out, her tailbone was fractured and took about six weeks for it to heal before she was able to come in to see if she needed an adjustment.

I enjoyed helping the patients of this medical doctor. I look forward to the day when all health-care professionals work together for the highest good of their patients.

Lower Legs and Feet

We have twenty-six bones in each foot, and we put a lot of stress on our feet. Many chiropractic techniques, including the Activator Method, address these subluxations.

When you think about the human body, it is quite an amazing design. The entire weight of the body goes down to the lower legs. The lower leg has two bones, the tibia and the fibula.

The fibula, the smaller of the two, is a non-weight-bearing bone used for muscle attachment. The lower end of the fibula is the "bump" we feel at the outer edge of our "ankle bone." A subluxation of the fibula can occur when you twist your ankle, causing a "posterior distal fibula" that responds to a chiropractic adjustment.

The other bone in the lower leg, the tibia, attaches to one bone in the foot and supports the entire weight of the body. That bone should be called the brother of Atlas, but instead, it is called the talus.

The talus, like Atlas, got its name from Greek mythology. Talus was a mechanical man built by Hephaestus, the only Greek god who was known to be born ugly. He was so ugly that his mother threw him off a cliff, breaking his legs. Hephaestus was a nice guy and became the god of blacksmiths, using volcanos to forge his man of steel.

Perhaps in an attempt to help him get around, he used his skills as a blacksmith to build a mechanical man named Talus. The bone in each foot that forms a joint with the tibia and supports the entire weight of our body was named after Talus.

The chiropractic problem I sometimes see is that the bone just in front of talus, called the navicular, sometimes "pops up" out of its normal position. No wonder. You would pop up, too, if you had all that pressure abutting you. Because of the extreme job it has, the navicular sometimes needs to be adjusted, relieving pressure in the feet.

Plantar Fasciitis – Subluxation of the Heel Bone

There are twenty-six bones in each foot. The largest bone in the foot is the calcaneus, or the heel bone.

A thick piece of connective tissue called the plantar fascia extends along the bottom of the foot and attaches to the heel bone. A subluxation of the heel bone causes stress on the place where the plantar attaches. This leads to inflammation and the painful condition known as plantar fasciitis.

In many patients I see with this problem, the direction of misalignment of the heel bone is usually superior. That is, the back of the heel bone is slightly tipped up, causing the stress on the place where the fascia is attached.

A subluxation of the calcaneus can occur when jumping and landing on the heels. This can cause the calcaneus to subluxate in a superior direction, causing undue stress on the place where the fascia attaches. This stress leads to inflammation and the plantar fascia becomes known as plantar fasciitis, because "itis" means inflammation.

Even if patients cannot remember jumping and landing on their feet, it is something most kids do at one time or another. It could be a long-standing subluxation of the heel bone that finally develops the symptoms of plantar fasciitis.

Symptoms of plantar fasciitis include pain on the bottom of the foot. It is usually worse first thing in the morning, upon taking the first steps out of bed. The cause of plantar fasciitis is stress at the place on the heel where the fascia attaches. Many times, a chiropractic subluxation of the calcaneus is the underlying cause of this problem.

And then there are the toes. Sometimes, perhaps from stooping down and bending your foot at the toes, or wearing high heels, the joints are stressed where the foot bones attach to the toe bones. The result is something called "dropped metatarsals." Dropped metatarsals are a subluxation that needs to be adjusted from the bottom of the foot. My patients with foot problems look forward to getting their feet adjusted.

Things to do to prevent foot problems include:

- Do not walk barefoot on hard floors. Feet need proper arch support. The only time to walk barefoot is on the bare earth, either the beach or grass.
- Picking up a towel with the toes is a good exercise for maintaining a healthy arch.
- For a good foot massage, roll the foot over a golf ball.
- Using a frozen plastic water bottle as a foot roller is a good way to relieve inflammation.
- Have your chiropractor evaluate if custom arch supports would be beneficial to you.

Chapter Fourteen
Posture

As a chiropractor, I am perhaps more aware of posture than most people. Paying attention to your posture and making a conscious effort to have your body in the best possible mechanical position have incredible benefits.

How you sit, how you stand, and how your head is lined up with your body as you perform your daily activities are important considerations that can affect the health of your body. I tell my patients to be aware and concerned about good posture in whatever task they are performing.

First and foremost, your skull should be perfectly aligned with the bones in the top of your neck. By doing so, the mental impulses from the brain can flow freely from the brain, down the spinal cord, and out to every cell and organ of your body.

Having your wrists higher than your hands for an extended period of time can cause subluxations in the bones of your arms and hands, causing symptoms of carpal tunnel syndrome.

Becoming aware of the position of your body as you perform daily activities is the first step in preventing problems. Repetitive motions that put too much stress on the joints of the body can cause damage to the nerves and joints.

Ergonomics

Ergonomics is a field of study that strives to figure out the best possible working environment for the frame of the skeletal system. It is the science that deals with making your workstation as biomechanically friendly to your body as it can be.

As a chiropractor, I appreciate ergonomics because it creates a work space that takes pressure off the joints of the body and helps the worker maintain a healthy posture while working. Some questions that are studied by those who practice ergonomics include:

- Is your desk chair at the right height so that your knees are equal or lower than your hips?
- Is the middle of your computer screen at eye level?
- As you type, are your wrists and hands in a flat, neutral position as they would be if your arms were hanging by your sides?
- Are you using your shoulder to move your mouse rather than exerting your wrist and hand?

- Do you have a lumbar support pillow? Are you sitting up straight so that you maintain a normal low back curve as you type?
- Are you relaxed while typing?
- Are you overreaching to move the mouse?

Before you type on your computer, make certain that your wrists are not too low in relation to the keyboard. Have your wrists as level and flat as possible in relation to your arms to prevent stress on the carpal tunnels while typing.

Is your laptop computer directly in front of your eyes? Do you have to tilt your head up or down to look at it? Can you make improvements to your workstation to improve ergonomics?

Sitting Is the New Smoking

Ever since it was discovered that smoking is bad for us, we have been told to quit smoking.

An Australian study published in 2012 in the *British Journal of Sports Medicine* compared sitting and smoking. We are now being told to quit sitting. Sitting is bad for us. According to the study, every hour we sit takes twenty-two minutes off our life. Actually, sitting is worse than smoking, because according to the study, smoking a cigarette only takes eleven minutes off our life.

I guess that each of us should get up right now, march in place a dozen times, and then sit back down. (I did!)

Ernest Hemingway stood at a podium to write. He did not know that sitting was the new smoking, but he suffered from back pain that made it impossible for him to sit for any length of time.

I visited his home in Key West, which is now a tourist attraction. Peeking into his writing room, I could see the podium where he stood to write. The advice I would have given him would include putting a little five- to six-inch block of wood on the floor and place one foot on it while writing to take the pressure off the sacroiliac joints. Also, I would have told him to stop writing every half hour or so to march in place ten to twelve times. Marching in place relieves pressure on the ligaments that connect the bones of the pelvis. And of course, I would have encouraged him to find a good chiropractor!

Forward Head Posture

Right now, you could be jutting your head forward to look at the computer screen or to look at this book. Those who spend time on their mobile devices are especially prone to developing forward head posture.

When it comes to bad posture, forward head posture is a common problem, because it leads to other postural distortions. To determine if we are suffering from forward head posture, we should have someone take a look at our posture while we are standing in a neutral position. I do this as part of my chiropractic exam.

There are two ways to examine the posture. The first thing I do is to look at my patient to see if one shoulder or hip is higher than the other or if the head is tilted to one side or the other. Then I look at the patient from the side.

Ideally, we should be able to draw an imaginary line from the ear, down through the shoulder, the hip, the knee, and the ankle. Most people, however, have some postural distortions. One of the most common postural distortions is the forward head posture.

Forward head posture can lead to other problems in the spinal column. For instance, when the head juts forward, the upper body moves backward and the hips move forward. As the body compensates for bad posture, we are on our way to creating subluxations that will need to be corrected with chiropractic care.

Forward head posture not only leads to neck and upper back tension and stress, but left unchecked, the chain of events due to compensations can lead to mid back pain, low back pain, loss of balance or dizziness, the development of arthritis, and crammed abdominal organs.

Just last night, I was watching a movie with my sister and brother-in-law. One of the characters in the movie was an elderly man with terrible posture. He was stooped over and his head was jutting forward. I commented on his bad posture.

"He needs an adjustment," said my brother-in-law.

My sister nodded her head in agreement. "He sure does."

I replied, "He needed an adjustment a long time ago."

Hold in Your Tummy

I would like to recommend that we all contract our abdominal muscles as much as we can and as frequently as we can throughout the day. "Holding in the stomach," as if preparing for someone who is going to punch us in the abdomen, is an isometric exercise in an area of our body that really needs it.

The central part of our body, our core, is a cylinder comparable to a tin can. If the tin can has a dent on one side, such as weak abdominal exercises, there is added stress to the other side of the can, which is our low back. Strengthening the core of our body reduces stress on the low back muscles.

In the first quarter of cadaver lab, the mission was to open the body and remove the organs. After removing the heart and lungs, it was time to open the abdominal cavity. The professor granted the privilege of performing the first incision to one of the guys in the class who was acting as if it was no big deal. Hoping I would not faint, I was amazed at how much stuff popped out. First of all, there was a ton of scrambled eggs that had to be removed, which, I soon found out, was fat. But even when the fat was gone, there was so much stuff—intestines, gall bladder, liver, but mostly intestines. I wondered how a surgeon would ever get all that stuff back in after an operation.

My point is that the abdominal organs are really crammed into our abdominal cavity. If you slump forward or do not stand up or sit up straight, you add to the cramming of our abdominal organs, thereby reducing their ability to function properly. You want those organs to work as efficiently as possible. Sitting up straight, head back, shoulders back are favors we should all do for ourselves.

A man who lived in Nashville visited the Parthenon in Greece and fell in love with the structure. He came back to the United States and was inspired to build a replica of the Parthenon in Nashville. That is amazing in itself, but when you step inside, even more amazing is that you will see a fifty-foot statue of Athena.

Watch Your Neck

Inside this Parthenon there are benches perpendicular to Athena, so you can sit down, turn your head toward her, and look up to stare at the magnificent sculpture. I do not recommend turning your head and looking up at anything. Looking up to see something towering fifty feet above your head in close quarters is stressful on your neck.

If you ever get the chance to visit something as magnificent as Athena, be aware of bending, twisting, and turning your head. If I ever visit Athena again, I will bring my yoga mat and ask the manager on duty for permission to lie down on the floor. From a nice, relaxed repose, I will gaze at this masterpiece without putting my neck at risk of getting a subluxation.

Becoming aware of posture and doing whatever you can do to improve your posture are the first steps in making positive changes in the way you can position your body for any activity you do.

Considering the ergonomics of your workstation and making any necessary improvements will help the biomechanical alignment of your body. Sometimes, only a small change is needed to make a big difference. Minimizing the risk of subluxation is a goal worth achieving. Anything we can do to prevent the degeneration of our spinal column will pay off in health dividends in the years to come.

Chapter Fifteen
Stress Management

Most times, stress is related to the thoughts we think. Unpleasant thoughts lead to unpleasant feelings. These unpleasant feelings affect our nervous system, causing the release of stress hormones such as adrenalin and cortisone. A constant stream of these chemicals causes subluxations.

Nervous Tension

One afternoon, sitting in my office, I answered the phone to hear an elderly woman calling.

"Do you treat nervous tension?"

As a chiropractor, I don't give "treatments," I give adjustments. I don't try to explain that to them right away, because it may confuse them. But it's true, I don't give "treatments," I give adjustments.

- Treatments come from outside the body.
- Treatments treat symptoms.
- Chiropractors correct the cause of the symptoms.

- An adjustment turns on the natural healing power of the body.
- The body heals from the inside out.

Rather than try to explain all that to her on the first phone call, I asked her a few questions, such as,

"Have you ever been under chiropractic care before?"

She said no, a friend urged her to give me a try.

"What kind of symptoms are you having?" I asked, wondering what she meant by nervous tension.

"I'm just so nervous all the time. I feel shaky. I have a lot of nervous tension."

I told her that I would be happy to meet with her and do a brief chiropractic exam to see if she had a chiropractic problem.

During our first visit, I learned that she was in her late seventies. Blood pressure medication was keeping hypertension under control.

Taking her case history, I found out that she had an automobile accident many years ago. From what I was hearing, it sounded to me as if she could have used a chiropractor earlier in her life.

I explained how the trauma she suffered could have caused minor misalignments of her skeletal system. I explained to her that I would be finding and correcting minor misalignments of her spinal column, which would take pressure off the nervous system.

During the chiropractic exam, I palpated the muscles surrounding her spinal column. The muscles in her back were in a constant state of contraction.

They felt stiff and hardened. Then I did a leg length check and some preliminary isolation reflex testing. I could see she had many subluxations of her spinal column that needed to be adjusted.

I suggested that we give it a two or three visits before deciding if chiropractic was going to work for her. I told her that sometimes I am quite surprised when someone such as herself, who has never had an adjustment in her life, responds quite well to chiropractic care.

I took a plastic model of the spine and placed it on my adjusting table. Demonstrating how I was going to adjust her, she agreed that a chiropractic adjustment sounded like a good idea.

In her case, I only made a few adjustments on the first visit. I knew that once the interference to the nerves to her muscles was reduced, tight muscles would begin to relax and lactic acid would be released. I did not want her to feel sore afterward.

I told her that drinking extra water and taking some deep breaths to get oxygen to the muscles would be helpful.

When I saw her at the follow-up appointment, she was feeling much better. She seemed more relaxed and said she was telling her friends about me.

"It's amazing," she said. "I never believed in chiropractic, but I do now."

Grumpy Patients

It's amazing to me how grumpy some people can be when they don't feel good. On the bright side, it's just as amazing to see how much their personality improves when they begin feeling better.

When I get grumpy patients, I know they are probably grumpy because they do not feel good. Sometimes, when patients come back for a follow-up visit feeling much better, I hardly recognize them. Not only do they feel better, but they look better.

I say, "You look better today!" Although, what I really want to say is, "You're not as grumpy as the last time I saw you." ☺

Learning to Relax

Learning to relax and quiet the mind is a skill worth learning. Learning to relax takes time and practice, but it is a skill that will provide benefits to you for the rest of your life. It can be compared to learning to play a musical instrument.

1) Lie down and make yourself comfortable. Place a pillow under your knees to take pressure off the low back and a small pillow under the neck, if desired.

2) Begin by taking a breath in through your nose and exhaling through the nose. As you inhale, feel your abdomen rise. This ensures that the breath is full and complete rather than just a shallow breath.

3) Begin using your mind to relax your body by saying to yourself, "My left arm is heavy." Then, "My right arm is heavy." Giving these mental instructions to your body does two things: First, it instructs the muscles to release and let go. Second, it gives your mind something else to think about rather than the worrisome thoughts you may be thinking.

4) Proceed through every part of your body, making your body feel heavy. Very, very heavy…

5) Next, beginning again with the left arm, use your mind to give your body instructions to make each body part feel warm. "My left arm is warm… My right arm is warm." When you get to your toes, your entire body will feel warm and heavy…and very relaxed.

6) If your thoughts drift off to other things, simply take note of the thought. Then return your thoughts to your breathing. Become totally aware of your breathing. Observe yourself inhaling and exhaling. See your breath as a healing, soft, pink light coming into your body. See your breath leaving your body as gray tension being released.

7) If something from the past is causing your stress, use your breathing to release the past. As you inhale, breathe in a wonderful new future. As you exhale, release the past.

Learning to relax the body and quiet down your internal chatter leads to better health and well-being.

Breathing and Stretching

When we breathe and exhale, not all of the air comes out of our lungs. Some air is left in the bottom of the lungs. This stale air is known as the "tidal reserve volume." I think it is a good idea to get a full exchange of air at least once a day, preferably in the morning. Exhale normally, and at the end of the exhalation, force yourself to exhale a little more. You will be amazed at how much more air comes out.

Taking a series of deep breath does many good things for you:

- It oxygenates the blood so that the blood going to our brain contains more of what it needs.
- Breathing oxygenates muscles, and because muscles need oxygen to relax, breathing deeply helps to relax the muscles.
- Breathing gives us something to think about other than our worries and concerns.
- Breathing connects us to the power within us.
- Taking ten deep breaths is a great way to begin the day.

If learning to relax seems impossible or difficult, I recommend that my patients see a mental health counselor. My current practice is located in an office with mental health counselors. I refer patients to them who have emotional, stress-related issues. Working together with other health professionals to achieve the best possible results for my patients is my vision and my goal.

Many people have not had enough training for learning how to deal with stress. Some people are born with a calmer, more serene nature than others. But for a lot of us, managing stress is an ongoing process. Professional counselors are experts when it comes to helping people handle the stress in their lives.

Chapter Sixteen
Food for Thought

The United States Department of Health and Human Resources reports that sixty-four percent of all Americans are overweight or obese, and that the percentage is on an upward trend. They also report that deaths by poor diet and lack of exercise rose thirty-three percent in one decade and may soon overtake tobacco as the number one preventable cause of death.

The Standard American Diet

The Standard American Diet is **SAD**. Fast food, junk food, diet sodas, which I call "chemical cocktails," sugar-filled drinks, and processed factory substances we mistake for food are all part of the problem.

Many cases of diabetes, heart disease, cancer, high blood pressure, and obesity are directly related to diet and lifestyle. It's been said that up to eighty percent of all diseases are diet and lifestyle related.

Improving our diets can improve our health and prevent diseases associated with diet. Becoming aware of the food we eat and the drinks we drink are the first steps toward making positive changes.

A Google search for "books on what to eat" produces 589,000 findings. Yikes. That's a lot of books! And a lot of rules! The selection of diet books available leaves us wondering, "What are the best food choices for me and my family? Should we eat high-fat, low-fat, or no-fat foods? Who knows? Is one diet good for everyone? How are we supposed to figure it all out?

We just can't ignore the subject of diet, because we have to eat. Bombarded with advertisement, we couldn't ignore the topic even if we tried.

Tantalizing television commercials, billboards, yummy-smelling movie theater popcorn, shopping mall food courts, grocery stores, fast-food restaurants, gas station snack shops, strategically placed vending machines, and other convenient ways to buy something to eat entice us at every turn. But are we choosing to eat the foods that are best for us?

Got Meat?

Whether or not humans are supposed to eat meat is an interesting and controversial subject. No one knows for sure.

Genesis says, "Behold, I have given you every plant yielding seed which is upon the face of the earth, and every tree with seed in its fruits and you shall have those for food."

Later in the Bible, Noah was told he could eat anything he could find, including animals.

In 1906, *The Jungle*, a book by Upton Sinclair, was published. In his book, readers were told about the horrible working conditions of immigrants working in the meat-packing industry. *The Jungle* brought attention to the working conditions of the meat-packing industry. As a result, laws were created to protect the workers. Interestingly, that book is still in print today, 107 years later!

Today, the concern is not so much about the way the workers are treated. It is about the way the animals are treated.

Oprah Winfrey was sued by the cattle industry for saying that she would never eat another hamburger after she became aware of what happens in the cattle industry. No one sued Albert Einstein when he said, "Nothing will benefit human health and increase the chances for survival of life on earth as much as the evolution to a vegetarian diet."

Paul McCartney didn't get sued when he said, "If anyone wants to save the planet, all they have to do is stop eating meat. That's the single most important thing you can do. It's staggering when you think about it. Vegetarianism takes care of problems including ecology, famine, and cruelty." Paul McCartney and his daughter have established a Web site promoting the idea of "meatless Mondays."

Meatless Mondays

A Meatless Monday campaign is being promoted as a good way to improve diet and health by starting off the week on a healthy note. It is based on the fact that incorporating more plants into your diet are better choices for your long-term health.

The first Meatless Monday began during WWI, when the United States Food Administration (USFA) tried to get people to conserve food. President Woodrow Wilson helped promote the idea by printing recipes and meal-planning ideas.

Then in WWII, Meatless Monday was promoted again as meat became rationed. The media helped the effort by printing magazine articles and books that featured meals without meat.

Once again, Meatless Monday is an idea that is sweeping the country. State governments, schools, and even restaurants are supporting the idea. This time, though, rather than to conserve food, Meatless Monday is designed to improve health. Although Meatless Monday is an idea that originated in the United States, the campaign is extending to countries across the globe. Some countries, such as the Netherlands, are trying to expand on the idea by establishing a Vegetable Thursday.

Lab-Produced Meat

An August 2013, it was reported that scientists in the Netherlands produced a hamburger in a laboratory from cow stem cells. They invited members of the media to a press party for a taste. They told the reporters that developing countries are getting richer and are going to want more meat. They said meat grown in a laboratory would be a good way to meet (no pun intended) the growing demand.

The cofounder of Google presented researchers with a grant to keep doing this sort of research. Maybe this will settle the argument between vegetarians and meat eaters, although now, Jewish people have something to debate: Will this hamburger grown in a laboratory be kosher?

Another food idea in the news recently was a United Nations report suggesting humans should eat more insects to meet the need for food. They are high in protein and easy to grow. To me, a hamburger grown in a laboratory is more appealing. Although it makes me wonder, what's wrong with rice and beans? They are cheap, easy to transport, a complete protein, and healthy.

Food Choices

The best guidance we can get regarding what diet we should follow is the guidance we receive from within. The innate intelligence of our body will tell us what foods are good for us and what foods to avoid.

The only way to know for sure if we are supposed to eat meat is to see how we feel while eating it and how we feel after eating it.

Our thoughts and attitudes toward the food we eat also play a role in determining if a food choice is a good one. How we feel about the food we eat is a contributing factor as much as the food itself.

A relaxed attitude while eating allows our digestive system to work efficiently. Feeling badly about our food choices can affect the way our body reacts to the food we eat. If we are anxious about our food choices, the mental stress causes a reaction in our nervous system that prevents food from being digested easily.

The Shellfish Story

One of the most intriguing topics of discussion my biochemistry professor covered in chiropractic college was the idea of transmutation. He said that our body has the capability of changing one molecular structure into another depending upon the needs of the body. He told us that our bodies are like chemical factories. There are millions, perhaps billions, of chemical reactions that occur in our body at any given moment.

This process of transmutation makes up for the fact that our diet may not be perfect. He said we can make molecules we need from the molecules that are available. We shouldn't take that to mean that we shouldn't pay attention to the fact that some foods are better for us than others, but we needn't stress out quite so much about all the different rules because the human body can adapt to what we eat.

Experiments in Paris by French chemist C. Louis Kervran prove that shellfish make themselves a new shell in one day in water that has no calcium. This is quite amazing because when the body of the crab is analyzed for calcium, it was found that the crab only had enough calcium in its body to make about three percent of the shell. Yet, when taken out of seawater and placed into water that has no calcium, the crab was able to make itself a complete new shell.

GMOs

GMO stands for genetically modified foods, and this is one of the latest issues facing those who want to eat healthy. In creating GMO foods, scientists take the genes from the DNA of one species and force them into another species to create a food that is easier for farmers to grow. The benefits of GMO foods for the farmers include crops that can repel weed killers and bugs. The biggest GMO crops are soy, corn, and sugar beets.

One of the first GMO experiments was done by taking an antifreeze gene from the DNA of an Arctic fish and injecting it into the DNA of a tomato to see if the tomato could then withstand freezing temperatures. From there, it was discovered that crops could be genetically modified to withstand weed killers.

Today, most of the corn and soybeans we eat have been grown with genetically modified seeds, and people across the world are debating the issue.

Some say that GMOs are okay for us. Others say that GMOs are "Frankenfood" and cause health problems for us. Who knows for sure? But the opposition to GMOs has forced many countries in Europe to ban the use of genetically modified food in their food supply. In the United States, our FDA does not require food manufacturers to label foods as containing GMO products, but Connecticut is on the way to becoming the first state to pass laws regarding the use of genetically modified foods.

A Google search on genetically modified foods gives over twenty-four million results, and with that much information out there about GMOs, I could write about it till the organic cows come home. But it's up to each of us to investigate the issue and teach our children about the issue so that when they grow up, they can address these serious issues for themselves and their families.

The questions, controversies, and arguments for and against what we should eat are a huge issue. The best you can do is to educate yourself and take appropriate action to ensure the health of yourself and your loved ones.

Chapter Seventeen
Think for Yourself

Tuned into our computer or mobile device, listening to the radio or television, we are bombarded with information from the outside world. Listening to the opinions of others, telling us what they think we should do and what we should not do, sometimes drowns out what our inner guidance system is telling us is the right thing for us to do.

With so much information coming at us from so many directions and from so many people, it's sometimes rather difficult to hear what our innate intelligence is telling us what to do, yet the most reliable source of guidance we have is the guidance that comes from within.

"Whatever You Do, Don't Go to a Chiropractor!"

I heard that bit of advice while attending a networking event and meeting a woman who had been in an accident and was suffering from neck pain. I told her I was a chiropractor and explained how I might be able to help her.

A person walked up and joined the conversation, but missed hearing the part about me being a chiropractor. Hearing about her accident, he told her, "Don't even consider going to a chiropractor."

The woman opened her eyes wide at this comment and looked at me to see how I would react.

I looked at him, smiled, and said, "I'm a chiropractor."

He stammered a bit and backtracked from his comment. From my point of view, people should be allowed to think for themselves.

Rather than tell someone to never go see a chiropractor, a better suggestion might be, "Don't go to a chiropractor if you don't feel good being around that particular chiropractor."

Would you agree with someone who told you, "Don't ever go to a surgeon"? Perhaps a more supportive approach might be, "Don't ever let a surgeon operate on you if you don't feel good being in the presence of that particular surgeon."

Tolerance for different ways of thinking could go a long way to create peace on the planet. Allowing others to make their own decisions according to the innate intelligence within them is probably a better way for humans to relate. Allowing others to be who they are and think what they want to think, as long as they are not harming anyone, could make this world a much better place.

We have a responsibility to ourselves to interview our health-care providers to see if they are the one we will hire to take care of us. Every doctor, whether he or she is a chiropractor or a medical doctor, is an individual with unique characteristics and unique personality traits. Every patient is different. You have the right and the responsibility to yourself to choose health-care providers you trust and who inspire you to feel comfortable in his or her presence.

"You Have to Keep Going Back"

Many people who make their way to a chiropractor for the first time are skeptical. They've heard stories that "once you go to a chiropractor, they make you keep coming back." I explain that common misconception in the following ways:

- When you get the oil changed in your car, do you keep going back to get the oil changed when it needs to be changed? Many people take better care of their car than their body, but you should take good care of your spine with regular checkups and adjustments if needed.
- Once you get your teeth cleaned, do you keep going back to get them cleaned again when they need it?
- Once you get an adjustment on your teeth by an orthodontist, do you keep going back for more adjustments?
- If a medical doctor gives you a prescription for ten pills, do you just take one?

Stages of Care

I consider my patients to be my partners in their health care. I work with them to come up with a care plan that fits their needs and desires. There are three basic types of chiropractic care, and education is important so that we can decide which care plan works best for them.

- **Relief care:** Everyone is different, and everyone has a miracle within. Some miracles are small and some miracles are huge. Some people get an incredible amount of relief with just one or two visits, and sometimes, it takes several adjustments to get relief. It is not uncommon for a chiropractor to adjust a patient two or three times a week for a week or two. I compare it to getting a prescription for a bottle of pills from the pharmacy. You don't just take one. You may have to take several for it to work for you.
- **Corrective Care:** Patients who understand the value of having a healthy spinal column for a healthy body continue to come in to get corrective care even after the symptoms are gone. Early detection and correction of a subluxation is a good idea, because the symptoms associated with a subluxation sometimes take time to appear.
- **Maintenance Care:** Many patients just want relief from their symptoms, so they come in

when they are in pain. After a visit or two, they go away until something happens and they feel they need another adjustment. Maintenance care is a good idea, because preventing a problem is often easier than fixing the problem. Maintaining the health of your spine is just as important as taking care of your teeth or your car.

The Chiropractic Lifestyle

When we're in our twenties, everyone seems pretty healthy and pretty much in the same general condition. When I get patients who are in their twenties, I know it will just take an adjustment or two to get them back on track. They don't have the degenerative changes in their spinal column that come with neglecting to take care of their spinal column.

It's later in life that the real difference can be seen between those who have been under chiropractic care and those who have not. It's amazing to me, and inspiring also, to meet patients in their eighties who have been under chiropractic care for most of their life. They are active, agile, and living their lives to the fullest. There are no dimmer switches turning down the power. The light within is shining brightly.

I remember one woman in her eighties who told me it was amusing for her to go to her medical doctor for checkups. She said the office staff would gather around to look at her as if she were a spectacle.

"They couldn't believe that at my age, I wasn't on any medication. Made me feel like an alien or something," she said with a laugh. She was proud of the fact that her chiropractic lifestyle kept her healthy.

Chapter Eighteen
Spinal Hygiene

Taking care of our spine is as important as taking care of our teeth. If our teeth decay, we can have dentures. If we neglect our spinal column and allow it to decay, replacements are not available.

Taking care of your spinal column is a wise preventative measure because the spinal column is home to your spinal cord. The spinal cord is the power line connecting our brain to our body. Maintaining a healthy relationship between the spinal nerves and the bones of the spinal column keeps the body functioning at 100 percent.

If there was a user's manual that came with the human body, it would include information regarding the care and maintenance of the human frame. It would include information that would help the occupant of the body understand how their magnificent body is held together.

Ligaments

We have 206 bones in our body, and these bones are connected to each other by ligaments. Ligaments are somewhat like thick rubber bands that give a little. When we do stretching exercises, we stretch the ligaments to the end of the normal range of motion, which helps keep the joint flexible.

Muscles and Tendons

Muscles taper off at each end and become tendons. Tendons attach the muscles to the bones. When the muscle contracts, it pulls on the tendon and the bone moves. Whereas ligaments hold the bones together, muscles move the bones.

Sprains and Strains

A sprain happens when a ligament gets stretched too far beyond its normal range of motion and is usually the result of physical trauma. When a muscle gets worked too hard, we call it a strain.

Sprains and strains are the result of pushing the body too hard, either intentionally or accidentally.

I have patients involved in automobile accidents come to me as soon as possible after the accident to get checked for subluxations. I believe that patients who are under chiropractic care are less prone to injuries from minor accidents. On the other hand, if someone is subluxated and gets into an accident, the injuries could be worse.

Tendonitis

Tendonitis develops when the tendon that attaches the muscle to the bone gets overworked and becomes inflamed. The tendon is the part of the muscle that attaches to the bones. Working the muscle too hard puts excess stress on the tendon without giving the tendon a chance to rest, heal, and get stronger after heavy or repetitive use.

Itis means inflammation, and the best remedy for inflammation is rest combined with short applications of an ice pack. Ten minutes an hour is good. More than that will invoke the body's response to cold and the blood vessels will dilate in an attempt to send heat to the area, which is just the thing we are trying to control in an injury.

Trainers who work with professional athletes understand the importance of short periods of ice. They found that besides ten minutes per hour of ice, another five minutes of ice after thirty minutes will not invoke the heating response. So it's ten minutes at the top of the hour, and if desired, an additional five minutes on the half hour.

Whatever You Do, No Heat!

The innate intelligence of the body produces inflammation to protect the body from further injury. Inflammation causes swelling. Swelling restricts movement, preventing further injury.

Most of us are not going to continue playing tennis after spraining an ankle. We do not need excess swelling to tell us to give it a rest. Although I did hear a trainer for a professional basketball player tell the story of how the player sprained his ankle during a champion series game. The trainer said they kept the basketball player in the training room all night, placing ice on the ankle ten minutes at the top of the hour and five minutes at the bottom of the hour. By the next morning, it was as if the injury never happened. The player went out, played a starring role, and helped his team win the championship game.

That is in sharp contrast to the time I suffered a whiplash in a car crash when I was working as a newspaper reporter. As I said in the beginning of the book, it happened on my way home from work. My accident happened on a Friday and I spent the entire weekend with a heating pad on my neck. By Monday morning, I could not lift my head off the pillow. Looking back, I would have been much better off using ice in short increments. But now I know, and now you know, too.

The first step in the process of inflammation is that the blood vessels dilate so that white blood cells can be transported to the injured area. Since white blood cells fight infection, they would be needed if there was an open wound that could possibly become infected. In a sprain or strain injury, the dilated blood vessels are not needed. Reducing the swelling is desired because that is the natural process of healing. Applying cold to a soft tissue injury helps the blood vessels to contract. This reduces swelling and pain, and speeds up the healing process.

Taking Care of the Adjustment

But there are things you can do to "take care of your adjustment" and prevent chiropractic problems from happening in the first place. Here are some helpful hints you can use:

- Use ice on injuries ten minutes per hour, three to four times a day. Using heat on injuries increases inflammation.
- For men, thick wallets should not be carried in the back pocket because it creates a wedge under one side of the pelvis, leading to subluxation of the sacrum and pelvis, and low back pain. Consider carrying a smaller wallet that can be carried in the front pocket.
- For women, carrying a heavy purse on one shoulder causes an imbalance in the biomechanics of the skeletal system and leads to subluxation. Decide what things you really need to lighten the load.
- When lifting an object, be sure you are squarely facing what you lifting.
- When lifting, use your legs, not your back. This means bending your legs at the knees.
- Do not twist, bend, and exert at the same time. Reaching into the backseat of a car while sitting

in the front seat is a common mechanism of injury to the low back.
- When vacuuming or sweeping, keep the broom or vacuum close to your body. Never bend, twist, and exert.
- Never lift an object higher than your head.
- When lifting something from the floor, bend your knees and keep the object close to your body. Never bend from the waist to lift something. Squarely face the object being lifted.
- Hold objects close to your body when carrying them.
- Don't carry anything you can't handle with ease.
- Keep your head in line with your spine when sitting, standing, or lying in bed.
- Sleep on your side with knees bent, or on your back with a pillow under the knees.
- Be aware of your posture. Keep head high, chin slightly tucked, pelvis tucked.
- Don't sit in a chair where you have to turn your head or body to watch television or talk to someone. Adjust your seating accordingly so you are facing what you are watching.
- Sit in chairs low enough that allow feet on the floor, knees higher than hips. A small bench may be used to support the feet to accomplish this.
- Don't sit for more than thirty minutes at a time.
- Get at least thirty minutes of exercise four to five times a week. Walking is best. Consult

your physician before starting any exercise program.

- For weight training, the older we get, the more time is needed to allow our muscles to recover. Depending upon how strenuous the workout, you need to allow your body to recuperate between workouts of muscle groups. The amount of time it takes muscles to recover between workouts depends upon the age of the person and the intensity of the workout. Personally, I think two to three days between workouts of a muscle is a good recovery time, especially as we get older.

- Drink enough water to keep yourself hydrated and to flush out lactic acid produced by muscle contraction.

- Take a ten-to-fifteen minute time-out to relax and breathe when feeling fatigue during the day.

- Prepare for sleep by staying calm and quiet before going to bed.

- Limit watching the news. Worrying about things we have no control over causes anxiety and stress.

- For foot pain, roll the foot on an unopened can of food. Or freeze a small water bottle and roll the foot on the bottle. You can also roll your foot on a golf ball to give yourself a good foot massage.

- Learn to quiet the mind so that you can relax.

- Have your favorite inspirational reading handy to feed your mind positive thoughts.
- Find what makes you happy and spend time each day doing what makes you happy.
- Count your blessings.
- Don't take anything personally.
- Always do your best.
- Expect a miracle!
- Breathe.
- Get regular chiropractic checkups.
- Be happy.

Laughter

Can you laugh when there is nothing to laugh about, just for the sake of laughing? Can you call someone on the phone and leave them a laughing message just for fun? I love doing that! Can you wake up in the morning and laugh just because you woke up? Can you think of a good joke or remember a funny experience that makes you laugh?

There are "laughing clubs" popping up across the country. People are getting together to laugh because laughing is fun. And laughter is good for you. It has been said that laughing is "internal jogging."

I give away a little bimonthly chiropractic magazine called *Voice for Health* to my patients that includes interesting stories and information about chiropractic care. To my delight, there is a page of jokes. When the package of magazines arrives at my office every two months, I turn to the joke page first, where I find cute jokes to pass along to my patients.

Question: What kind of coffee did they serve on the *Titanic*?

Answer: Sanka!

A man goes to see his psychiatrist and says, "Doc, I think I am a deck of cards."

The doc says, "Go have a seat in the waiting room; I'll deal with you later."

I like making patients chuckle. I have a file folder filled with my favorite jokes. I like telling little jokes because I like to see my patients smile.

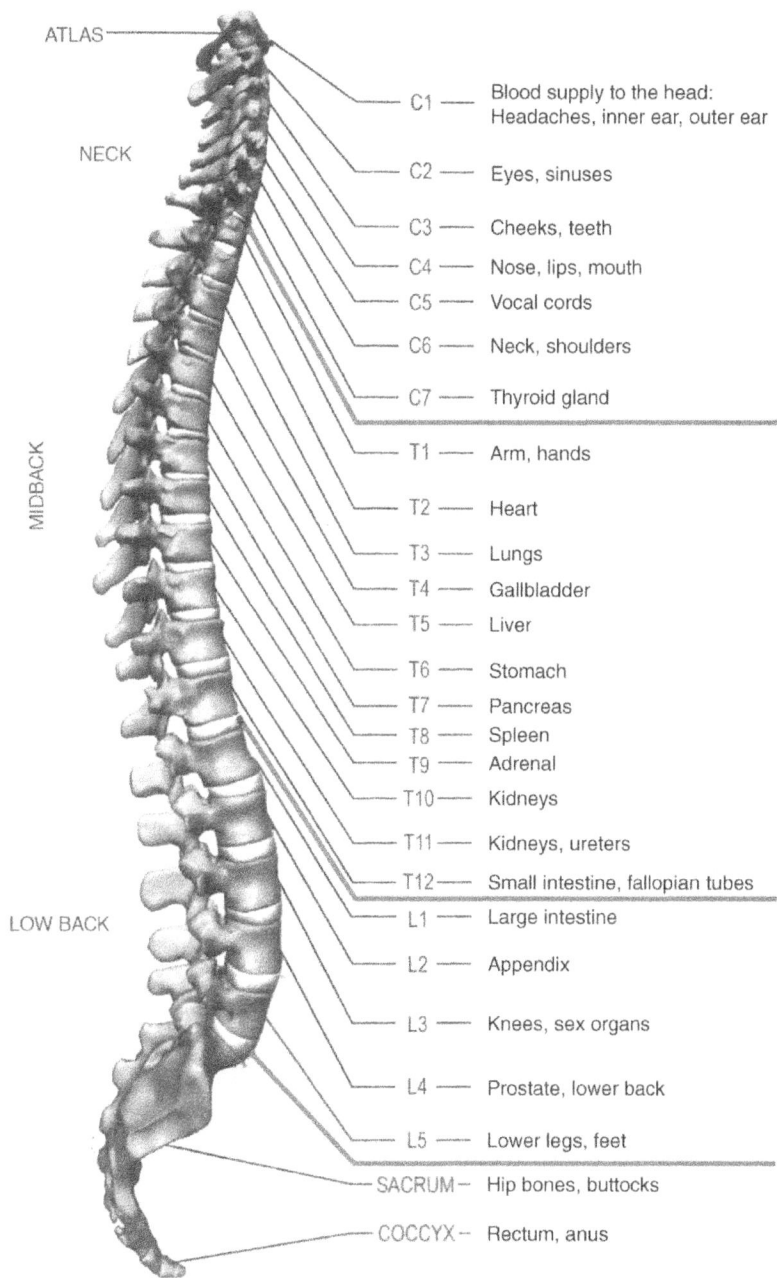

ATLAS

NECK

MIDBACK

LOW BACK

C1	—	Blood supply to the head: Headaches, inner ear, outer ear
C2	—	Eyes, sinuses
C3	—	Cheeks, teeth
C4	—	Nose, lips, mouth
C5	—	Vocal cords
C6	—	Neck, shoulders
C7	—	Thyroid gland
T1	—	Arm, hands
T2	—	Heart
T3	—	Lungs
T4	—	Gallbladder
T5	—	Liver
T6	—	Stomach
T7	—	Pancreas
T8	—	Spleen
T9	—	Adrenal
T10	—	Kidneys
T11	—	Kidneys, ureters
T12	—	Small intestine, fallopian tubes
L1	—	Large intestine
L2	—	Appendix
L3	—	Knees, sex organs
L4	—	Prostate, lower back
L5	—	Lower legs, feet
SACRUM	—	Hip bones, buttocks
COCCYX	—	Rectum, anus

Recommended Reading

What Your Doctor Never Told You – Dr. Jerry Zelm

The Power of Self-Healing – Dr. Fabrizio Mancini

Chiropractic First – Dr. Terry Rondberg

The Index to Chiropractic Literature – (a free Web site)

Contact the Author

To order additional copies of this book or to contact the author, please visit

DrFranAddeo.com

www.ingramcontent.com/pod-product-compliance
Lightning Source LLC
Chambersburg PA
CBHW030015290326
41934CB00005B/342